Hospice Nursing

Hospice Nursing

AN INTIMATE GUIDE

• • •

Margaret R. Crawford, BSN

ISBN-13: 9781546702252
ISBN-10: 1546702253
Library of Congress Control Number: 2017908032
CreateSpace Independent Publishing Platform
North Charleston, South Carolina

*There is no greater gift of charity you can give
than helping a person to die well.*[1]

—Sogyal Rinpoche

1 Sogyal Rinpoche, *The Tibetan Book of Living and Dying* (San Francisco: Harper, 1993), 186.

Contents

Acknowledgments

● ● ●

MY FIRST THOUGHTS OF GRATITUDE go to all the patients and families I have ever been with throughout my nursing career. Each patient, on some level, has shared something personal with me. I feel grateful hospice patients and families had the courage to ask for help at this profound time in their lives. I promised many who have already died that I would mention them in this book. They appear anonymously throughout. My heart swells remembering them. I thank them all for helping me grow. A few probably guessed I could use it.

Very deep and everlasting gratitude to the hospice I worked in. Incredible administrators, nurses, health aides, office staff, and one doctor work tirelessly every day and night (hospice care is not a 9–5'er) to give people the most meaningful and comfortable experience possible at the end of their lives. There are too many loving people at the hospice to name, but you all know who you are. I thank you for managing me so patiently.

Deep thanks to two outstanding friends, Deb and Michaelanne, both lifetime social workers/therapists, who read and squeezed out "ands" and rinsed away a thousand commas for me and you. They helped me revisit and revise. I know their hearts went into it because they are not capable of giving less than that.

Thank you always to my twin sister, Jane, and patient partner, Roger, who always have my back and strangely never seem to tire of it—at least not that I am aware of.

Thank you to Barbara Welch for her persistence and belief in what I set out to do.

Thanks to many patients, friends, and teachers who encouraged me to write at all.

Thank you, Dad, for encouragement long ago and for loving "whirds." Thank you, Mom.

I am beyond grateful.

Introduction

● ● ●

When I returned from a week vacation my boss called me to her office. "One of your patients has asked you not to return. They were uncomfortable with you and your approach." The irony was that I had begun to write about how extraordinary it is to be a hospice nurse while on the plane home. Reader, you may wonder why you should continue reading about hospice nursing from this author. On the other hand, you may feel relieved by my fallibility.

I wondered if I had a leg to stand on to write a book about hospice nursing. In the weeks following the dismissal, I immersed myself in my habitual quagmire of self-flagellation, thinking I should probably be a farmer, safe in my fields, keeping company with a few sweet-eyed, nonjudgmental animals, but I changed my mind. I realized I wanted to share the experience by writing this book. Hospice nursing is a mixed bag of highs and lows. Fortunately, the discomfort does not outweigh the succor we provide to our patients and their families or the compassion we experience as we give to and guide others. Hospice nursing gave me the opportunity to grow up.

I write about my trials and travails in hospice nursing hoping to spare you some of the discomfort, relieve you of having to eat crow too often (though some crow is good, and yes, it probably tastes like chicken), and to help you be a more informed, centered, confident nurse as you attempt to guide families and patients through life's end. Just hoping to spare you some time, possible humiliation, and pain. Why put your patients or your-self through your mistakes when I've gone through them for you? Thomas Edison said, "I have not failed. I've just found ten thousand ways that won't work." Allow me, dear nurse, to test the ten thousand ways.

If one of the goals for the book is to spare you some discomfort, neck and neck for goals is the hope for improved patient care. With just a bit more information provided from my experiences, maybe you will be able to give better care than I did. People might die more peacefully in your care. And that is so vitally important for everyone involved.

To reach this goal, I first delve into a few qualities and habits that I have found helpful over time, trial, and error. I discuss mental and emotional strategies, the inner work that I feel is helpful in this process, and I spend time on the outer work, the nonclinical how-tos of hospice care.

CHAPTER 1

Foundation of Hospice Care

● ● ●

GROWTH OFTEN COMES THROUGH ADVERSITY. Only occasionally does it arise from a pleasant experience. I find I benefit from scheduled doses of the former. Subconsciously I might even be the scheduler. I regularly made mistakes as a hospice nurse, and it was an awful feeling, embarrassing, all those words implying major squirm. However, I also know that being comfortable is not generally a condition from which expansion and creativity spring forth. Like the lotus growing from the mud, sometimes I need to get stuck in the mud, that fertile place, to learn my lessons. I am not claiming to be a beautiful lotus, but I do admit to my mud. Thich Naht Hanh is known to say, "No mud, No lotus." The experience of rejection became the inspiration and root experience from which many ideas in this book sprouted. It encompassed so many important lessons; for example, how to approach people, how to listen, when to back off, how to handle rejection, how to involve the team, and how to manage medication and pain management as well as discovering faith, working through pain, and finding humility. I generally feel fearless except when faced with rejection or annihilation.

The day I was thrown out, I didn't die. I benefited. I must add, this experience happened well into my tenth year working in hospice care and my twenty-seventh year of nursing.

Pema Chödrön said in her book *Start Where You Are*:

> We make a lot of mistakes. If you ask people whom you consider
> to be wise and courageous about their lives, you may find that they
> have hurt a lot of people and made a lot of mistakes, but that they
> used those occasions as opportunities to humble themselves and
> open their hearts. We don't get wise by staying in a room with all
> the doors and windows closed.[2]

Frederick Douglass said, "If there is no struggle, there is no progress." I
quote smart people often in the following pages. They say what needs saying so brilliantly.

If you are interested in my resume, read on, and if not skip, this short
paragraph. In my twenty-nine years of nursing I worked in OB/GYN,
medical-surgical, postpartum care, high-risk labor and delivery, adult
intensive care, a few years in the emergency room, and evolved into hospice ten years ago. Each field prepared me to blend into the next. There
is such similarity between labor and delivery and hospice care, but that
is a chapter I did not write. When I worked in the ICU, I felt relieved
when I removed the medical paraphernalia like tubes, cables, and drains
and turned off loud machines so that patients could die comfortably and
peacefully. I loved letting the patients and family make decisions. I loved
comfort care, and the more lenient drug doses allowed for symptom management. I was drawn to the gentleness of it all. I loved not forcing people
to live past their expiration dates. When I went into hospice care, I loved
doing things *for* people versus *to* them. In other settings, I often felt like
I inflicted discomfort, with little or no perceived benefit, on people who
felt powerless, angry, and afraid. As a hospice nurse, I had no moral issues
with my work.

---

2 Pema Chödrön, *Start Where You Are: A Guide to Compassionate Living* (Boston:
Shambhala, 1994), 184–185.

Respect

A hospice nurse practices and strives for a feeling of deep respect for people and is open to setting the highest intentions for their well-being. She also becomes aware of when she feels tempted to control someone's feelings, behavior, or decisions. As I developed this book, the focus seemed to revolve around respect for oneself and others, intention, and control—my letting go of it and patients and families' needing to maintain as much as possible.

I have heard it said that "Courtesy is the lubricant of society," and I feel respect is the lubricant of hospice care and the root of our work. This means we respect patient and family wishes, their decisions, where they are starting from, and where they want to end. We respect their living situations, their homes (gorgeous and not so much), their strange or estranged children and the reasons for it, their possessions, and their histories. We respect their intelligence, their education level, their faith, their level of cleanliness, and their pets. Their addictions. Their everything. We respect the lives these families have led without judgment. We respect ourselves for the above as well. We respect life and death, its process, and its timing.

This, of course, describes a perfect world with saintly nurses. Unsaintly nurses like me have daily opportunities to practice respect and release of judgment. We will have patients whom we fall in love with or feel an immediate connection with, and we enjoy them and their families immensely. And we will care for the seemingly unlovely people too. As nurses, we strive to treat everyone with equal respect and gentle care. You might be thinking "duh" to this, but when you are out there at the bedside of an unlovely and very difficult person, you might find yourself thinking otherwise.

Intentionality

Author Jon Kabat-Zinn says, "Intentions remind us of what is important. Intention informs our choices and our actions, our intentions serve as blueprints, allowing us to give shape and direction to our efforts and our lives."[3]

In order to set the highest intention for our patients and families, we must remove our opinions, agendas, and preconceptions about the homes we enter. Prominent nurse theorist Dr. Jean Watson, PhD, RN, said:

> When one declares intentionality toward an object or action, whatever resistance may be within tends to mobilize and dissipate, allowing manifestation of intention to be realized. Intentions do not refer to having a goal-directed outcome in mind, nor a specific purpose for directing another person or situation. Rather it is cooperating with the field, the emerging order, instead of trying to change it.[4]

The allowing can be a relief for those of us who tend to like having control. Hospice nursing will be a lesson in releasing control, and experiencing this cooperation with the Good Orderly Direction ('scuse me, but GOD) can be very beautiful.

One goal for a hospice nurse is to set an intention to be open to the evolution of the best outcome. There is a wonderful Reiki prayer that creates this open intention: "May we all be open to receive whatever it is we (or patient and family) need at this exact moment." We are regularly asked by patients and families, "How much time. What is going to happen?" As nurses, we can say we don't know, because we do not and cannot know how the best outcome will unravel. I was often surprised how well situations worked out for people, incredibly, without my intervention! A family

---

3 Jon and Myla Kabat-Zinn, *Everyday Blessings* (New York: Hyperion, 1998), 381.
4 M. Smith, "Caring and the Science of Unitary Human Beings," *Advances in Nursing Science* 21, no.4 (1999):14–28.

member would show up at the perfect time, the patient would die at the right moment. Not knowing is a relief. Death may seem to be the obvious outcome in hospice, but I believe the ultimate outcome is the family's experience and memory of the patient's dying process.

CHAPTER 2

Why Choose Hospice Nursing?

● ● ●

"Do ALL THE GOOD YOU can, in all the ways you can, by all the means that you can, to all the people and all the places you can, for as long as ever you can. Healing does not take place in the fast lane, nor does it take place as only stewarding the technical. For anyone called to the medical profession the true calling is this: access the healing gift we carry within."[5]

Jean Watson invites us to ask:

Why are we in this field (of nursing)? We are not just there to fix a body, diagnose, and treat. Healing is much more than that. It comes down thru the ages, from our ancestors and wisdom-traditions that call us into this work. And it is about honoring our very presence, our connectedness with another person in a given moment. And it is that caring moment that can actually be a critical turning point in my life, your life, and another person's life as we touch another person's humanity. What if we look at the foundation of our work? What if we honored the deep rich beauty of our humanity? It must again flourish because this is what healing is about.[6]

---

5 M. Stillwater and Gary Malkin, Angeles Arien in *Care for the Journey*, Companion Arts, 2005, CD-ROM #2.

6 M. Stillwater and Gary Malkin, Jean Watson in *Care for the Journey*, Companion Arts, 2005, CD-ROM #5.

It behooves nurses to inquire of ourselves why we choose to work with the dying. Hospice nurses should look at their experience with death, their feelings and fears, their personal and cultural perspective. We may have unfinished business regarding a death that was close to us. We may harbor guilt or anger over a close death. Your feelings about death (and life) will surely surface, and it will be helpful to prepare yourself. It is not helpful to become a basket case at the bedside of the dying or to avoid difficult bedside scenarios.

I think I chose hospice nursing because I love the intimacy of the work. I love the connection. Maybe I need the connection. Sometimes our inspirations are not altruistic. That's OK. We work with it. My dad had recently died when I started hospice nursing. Possibly I wanted to understand his process better. This was also my first exposure to home-care hospice, and I appreciated their services. There is not right or wrong reason to choose hospice nursing unless you are a drug-seeking Nurse Jackie (character in a TV show of that name about a high-functioning nurse addict that I became addicted to).

Jean Watson says:

> What if we realize that this is sacred work? And it is sacred because we are working with the life force of another as well as our own, on a shared journey. What if we pause and begin to realize that maybe this one moment, with this one person, is the very reason we are here on earth at this time?[7]

These words stuck in my memory, and I often think of them when I am with patients.

Watson says it so much better than I could:

> We are trying to return to the depths of our work. We know when we connect, even for a brief moment, we can feel much more

---

7 Stillwater and Malkin, *Care for the Journey*, #5.

purpose in our work. We know when this is missing we feel a void and we are dispirited. We also know patients feel the same. When we hold them in their wholeness we hold their healing for them and we help to sustain them when they are most vulnerable and we are also sustaining ourselves at the same time. This work is a spiritual practice. When we touch another person, we touch more than their body, we are touching their mind, their heart, their very soul. And when we look into the face of another person we look into the infinity and mystery of the human soul and when we look into the mystery and infinity of the human soul it mirrors the infinity and mystery back and into our soul and that is what connects us to this infinite field of universal love that we draw upon in our practices.[8]

Now, this describes a decent day in hospice nursing. There will be days when this image is not so clear. And the patient may be feeling the same about you too.

I love to look at the wedding or family pictures on the walls of my patients' homes and note their youthful, smiling eyes and relaxed posture, arms lovingly draped over their friends' or relatives' shoulders. In your mind's eye, place the photo as if it were a double exposure over the patient. Realize his or her humanity. A human life is a sacred thing regardless of our judgment. Connecting like this, transcending the physical, has the potential to transform your nursing practice. And we like transformation, right?

In casual, often brief conversations about hospice care, I am asked, "Isn't hospice depressing?" For me hospice work can be sad, but is not depressing. This is because we nurses can offer comfort and lighten the tremendous burdens patients and families experience. Alleviating symptoms, opening discussions, and assuaging fears allows more space for them to focus on

---

8 Stillwater and Malkin, *Care for the Journey*, #5.

nurturing one another and makes room for as much love as possible to freely flow. This is wonderful work. We sustain patients and families when they are most vulnerable.

People who are dying, and their families, need your expertise, experience, and compassion. Chogyal Rinpoche states in his book *The Tibetan Book of Living and Dying*:

> Peaceful death is really an essential human right, more essential perhaps even than the right to vote or the right to justice; it is a right on which, all religious traditions tell us, a great deal depends for the well-being and spiritual future of the dying person. There is no more charitable act than to help someone to die.[9]

I hope you will feel the great importance of the work you have chosen and appreciate the privilege and opportunity to be able to offer your gifts.

You will be rewarded in hospice work subtly, spiritually, and outwardly with warm feedback from patients and families. A patient's smile or giggle, his or her newfound comfort level, the relief the patient experiences because he or she (and the family) is being cared for by a professional, the patent's peaceful death, and the knowledge that you tried your hardest will inspire you. We are rewarded by witnessing the strength, love, and commitment of patients and families as they take on the enormous task of helping someone die at home even though they know nothing about how to care for someone who is dying. We are buoyed by their grit, grace, and bravery. We can emotionally escape the global condition, Washington, DC, and breaking Fox News just by being with these families. Seeing the best in people in their homes affirms the goodness in people. I am reassured that "love is all there is," as John Lennon said, and I feel spiritually uplifted.

---

9 Rinpoche, *The Tibetan Book of Living and Dying*, 186.

Hospice nursing offers opportunities for soul-searching and soul baring. It is a different species of nursing. If you have a history of working in units or on floors, this job will test you on different levels. I think every field of nursing has its own personality types that are drawn to it. Some of us move through a few of them before deciding where we function best. In hospice nursing we develop and use our wisdom, tact, diplomacy, creativity, and nursing knowledge. You will need to sit still at times, think outside the box, pray, and ponder what is best for folks. You will be challenged physically, emotionally, and mentally. Often, we need to think quickly for solutions without the benefit of having a colleague to call into the room for his or her opinion. In hospice nursing we have time to spend with people unlike in other fields of nursing. This is a huge benefit to both parties, and because of this I feel more is asked of the nurse emotionally. The hospice nurses I know love this aspect of their work.

Once in a while, experienced nurses will apply for a position at the hospice, and I have heard them say that they hope to retire here. They underestimate the amount of time investment needed, especially for case management. The paperwork alone will kill ya, to paraphrase Butch Cassidy as he jumped off the cliff. Prepare to be thinking about patients, charting, and making phone calls on behalf of your patients off shift. With time and experience, you will learn how to juggle it all, but don't be surprised if the work seems overwhelming in the beginning. Ask for support and spend time with the old-fogey nurses. Observe their survival techniques. This work is not for the nurse who has a tendency toward complacency or is seeking a cake job.

Hospice nursing differs a bit from hospital nursing. There are no shift buffers, meaning we don't have the varying perspectives from on-coming or off-going nurses and doctors. (Then again, there is no change-of-shift complaining.) There is no exchange of ideas on the spot. We don't have the camaraderie of being on the road all day. Because of this lack of exchange, many new and some old hospice nurses tend to worry endlessly into the wee hours of the night about possible flaws in their thinking and judgment. I have jumped out of bed long before the cat's 4:30 a.m. feeding to log into the hospice pharmacy to make sure meds will be delivered that day, or to write an e-mail to a coworker, or to gnash my teeth over something really dumb I said to a family member. We can feel burdensome responsibility, and this can erode our well-being. Our hospice chaplain offered this insight. "The RN does not own the patient and family; the patient and family belong to the team, working in collaboration with them." This does not have to be a lonely job because you do have the strength and intelligence of the team to bolster you. We all can become emotionally weary at times, so our self-care will be critically important. More on this later.

I am frequently informed by others that "I could not be a hospice nurse because I would get too attached." There is potential to become immersed in the patient's and family's experience, creating a blurry boundary with them. Over time we can learn the art of balanced giving and receiving. Nurses might be attracted to hospice nursing because of the implied intimacy of the work, the autonomy, and the knowledge that we can help people at a dramatic and sacred time in their lives. Some of us dive in wholeheartedly. We do our best and then some. We commit to people's peace of mind and comfort. And we try to do this for the fourteen other patients on our caseload. Over time, we attempt to learn how to give, how to step back, and how to let go and walk away. Sometimes the pendulum must swing to the side of weariness and sadness once too often to help us realize we can choose a different way to relate to these families.

We each have our challenges to meet, and some are more successful at this than others. I always admired the nurses who didn't bring it home at the end of the day. It was/is an ongoing challenge for me because it is in my nature to absorb more of others' experience than I need to. Call it what you will. Having it all together is not a prerequisite to writing this book or being a hospice nurse. I have tasks in this lifetime and learning to disengage from some people is one of them. Maybe that is another reason I went into hospice nursing. There is never one answer. Each nurse will have the opportunity to work on issues specific to him or her.

CHAPTER 3

First Things First

● ● ●

Self-Care

Our work and intention setting begins long before we knock on a patient's door. Our work must begin with ourselves (I know, you didn't want to hear that, but at least you don't have to get into small groups) so that we are instrumental in creating a healing environment for terminally ill people and their families. Self-respect and self-care are vital practices for nurses. We work on becoming healthy enough to be able to be open-hearted and insightful to people in intense, sometimes even chaotic, settings. We offer our calm and focused selves in homes and facilities with the intention of providing the best care possible. We offer optimum respect and dignity to all involved. This is only marginally possible if you are not up to snuff and unable to give from your heart. You can only give what you have, as we have heard countless times. For this reason, we need to know how to give gentle and loving attention to our own lives first.

Dr. Claudia Welch, a world-renowned teacher and practitioner of traditional Chinese medicine and Ayurveda and author of several books, told me she learned from her teacher that everything we bring into our lives—be it food, liquids, people, knowledge, and herbs—has either a medicinal, neutral, or poisonous effect. This means that we can strive to cultivate a medicinal effect on others. When we leave a patient's home, we want to feel assured he or she has benefited from our visit.

According to Dr. Welch, to benefit others we need to be able to deeply perceive our patients and families. From there, we may experience compassion, and then we can become the good medicine these families need. To deeply perceive, we must have our own sense of clarity and peace. Initially, I was disappointed to read this truth. I really like coffee, but I realized that when I am buzzed on coffee, or if I am concerned about anything other than what is in front of me, I am not in a condition to deeply perceive. I am into myself. A brain that is full of static or otherwise preoccupied is not in a receptive mode. I began to realize that to perceive deeply, one must be able to immerse oneself in the juice of moment. Then there is the capacity to feel with others, allowing a shared experience. This can be a very beautiful moment for you, the patient, and the family. It is not going to happen on a belly full of caffeine, if you are feeling preoccupied by your bad day, or you are under the influence of other harmful habits. Oh no. She isn't going to talk about harmful habits, is she? Not yet.

I spend a significant amount of time discussing self-care. I had to admit the truth of my unhealthy lifestyle habits to slowly learn how to care for myself so that I could interact in a sane and balanced way with others. If we agree with Jean Watson that nursing is a divine mission, then it benefits the nurse to become aware of his or her physical, emotional, and spiritual self. We have all heard the saying, "You can't pour from an empty cup" or "You can't give what you don't have." Ironically, in nursing there is a great deal of poor health due to stress, unhealthy lifestyles, and self-sabotaging habits. True self-care might be a brand-new and complex concept for some nurses, like it was for me. It can take years of unraveling many layers of our psychology to understand. My self-care was so poor for much of my nursing career, and though I may have thought I was functioning fairly well, certainly I was not. I am embarrassed by how unhealthy and immature I was. I know that now, at age fifty-nine, I continue to unmask what it means to deeply care for myself, and year by year I get a little stronger.

Self-care can be a mystery if one has been enmeshed in self-defacement as a way of life. It is easy to deceive ourselves in believing we take good care ourselves because the body is endlessly and ridiculously forgiving. I've heard it said that "youth hides all sin." We can abuse ourselves for a long time, but poor self-care will catch up to us. Dr. Welch quotes her teachers, "It is wise to live with reality, otherwise reality will certainly come to live with you."[10]

Even tiny attempts at self-care will instantly be rewarded because the body is so grateful for any love. It might even be starved for love. You might experience a few seconds of peace, a laugh at yourself, or renewed vigor and enthusiasm. Begin to fill your cup with sweet self-care. There are so many ways to do this that it is even a little exciting.

Dr. Deborah Zucker says:

> The way I see it, self-care isn't about the list of things you are sup-
> posed to do to be healthy or about keeping up with the new health
> fads or latest scientific theories. Self-care isn't about battling your-
> self into submission to satisfy the agendas of your inner critic.
>
> Self-care is about a fundamental orientation toward the self
> that is rooted in kindness and compassion. It is about nourishing
> all of who you are. And at its foundation, it is about your capacity
> to truly love and honor yourself and your life.
>
> As wonderful as all this sounds, true self-care is far from easy.
> The spiritual teacher Adyashanti often tells his students, "The
> person you'll have the hardest time opening to and truly loving
> without reserve is yourself. Once you can do that, you can love the
> whole universe unconditionally".
>
> So don't be surprised if self-care doesn't come naturally, or
> if you have unexpected and irrational resistance to doing it. We

---

10 Claudia Welch, DOM, *How the Art of Medicine Makes the Science More Effective: Becoming the Medicine We Practice* (Singing Dragon: London and Philadelphia, PA, 2015), 252.

all have baggage, wounds, traumas, and beliefs that keep us from being able to turn toward ourselves with the level of kindness, compassion, and loving care that we may easily be able to extend toward others."[11]

I encourage you to take an aerial view of yourself as you prepare to go to work. Perhaps you had a couple of glasses of wine last night or/and you have had two coffees already on an empty stomach. Maybe you woke up at 3:00 a.m. resenting the world. Perhaps a child or two or a mate irritated the bejesus out of you this morning with their spills and messes and the dog puked on the rug just before you left. You grab a half-pound stale bagel for breakfast and say to yourself, "I'll grab lunch later at Cumberland Farms." Maybe when you get in the car, you realize your shirt is on inside out and your socks don't match. I have done all the above, and I realized with embarrassment that if I were a patient or family member and saw me walk in the door, I might look past me hoping a real nurse was coming along behind. Step outside of yourself and be a witness to yourself, a hovering personal drone.

This can be a powerful experience. What I saw looking down was a woman who did not think much of herself. It was the jolt I needed to change the previously mentioned lifestyle habits that inhibited my being a nurse who could be present and helpful. I realized my patients deserved much better than a bleary, weary nurse, and this realization was pivotal to my nursing career. I started to clean up my act. If any of you watched *Nurse Jackie*, you realize how easily we can deceive ourselves.

"Self-observation brings us closer to truth. When the mind is steady, we can see a little truth. When the mind is disturbed, we can't see anything. Growth allows a portion of the mind to remain an objective witness even

---

11 Deborah Zucker, *The Vitality Map: A Guide to Deep Health, Joyful Self-care, and Resilient Well-Being,* (LomaSerena Press, 2016), 14.

in a disturbed state. The witness is always there, if one can keep a wakeful attitude in one's self" (Swami Kripalu, taken from a wall hanging at the Kripalu Center for Yoga and Health).

On a flight ten years ago I had an epiphany, another wake-up kick in the butt. The flight attendant was settling us for a flight. She hurried up and down the aisle, thin-lipped and unsmiling, stuffing bags in compartments, slamming the doors, grabbing blankets from empty seats. Though she might have been efficient, there did not seem to be any window to connect to her, nor did I have any desire. Instead, I wanted to keep clear of her energy. I had a dark aha moment, realizing I mimicked her movement frequently at work when I ran around the intensive care unit or emergency room focusing on machines and tubing and sadly not on the person in bed. I also saw clearly that I was not by any stretch creating a healing environment for my patients. I now thank this flight attendant for teaching me the lesson that my movement and body language, be it soothing, frantic, or anything in between, affects those around me.

I realized my patients needed calm. I needed calm. I needed to be calm.

ENERGY AWARENESS

Our families and patients subtly know the state we are in even if they would not be able to speak directly of it. Your health and state of mind leach out subtly to everyone you are in contact with. Recall the energetic field Jean Watson described. We are the pebble plunked into the lake whose reverberating ripples should be sweet and rhythmic, not sloshing, chaotic white caps.

Poet James W. Foley beautifully evoked the effects our words can have on in "Drop a Pebble in the Water: "Drop a word of cheer and kindness; just a flash and it is gone; But there's half-a-hundred ripples circling on and on and on, bearing hope and joy and comfort on each splashing, dashing wave; 'til you wouldn't believe the volume of the one kind word you gave."

Mother Teresa acknowledged the magnitude of this impact when she said, "Kind words can be short and easy to speak, but their echoes are truly endless."

The late Eknath Eswaran, renowned scholar, writer, and teacher at Blue Mountain Meditation Center in California, said in a discussion on YouTube. "A mind that is fast is angry, a mind that is slow is patient, still, loving."[12] Naturally, there are times when we need to move and act quickly in nursing. When I worked in the ER, a slow pace would not always benefit the patients, but there is a difference between frenetic and chaotic movement and quick yet purposeful and focused attention with the patient's needs being priority. The fast mind I believe Eswaran refers to is the distracted mind, the overly buzzed and unfocused mind. The caffeinated brain.

Jean Watson asks nurses to ask themselves, "Can I be present and really listen today to my patient?" If we feel balanced, we have more potential to connect with people. It is difficult to foster clarity and calmness when we are famished or have a liter of urine in our bladders. Anger, frustration, or preoccupation with a situation in your life will also weaken your on-point attention with your patients and families.

A devoted hospice nurse strives for optimum health not only for him-or herself, but for all those with whom he or she has contact. I do not claim to be perfectly healthy, but I am physically and emotionally healthier than when I started nursing. So much of life is a practice due to the ever-changing, nebulous state of, oh...everything. Optimal health is not something we simply achieve one day. It constantly fluctuates with the season, the time of day, our ages, and our situations at the time. We need

---

12 "The Training of Attention," Eknath Eswaran. Accessed 2010. www.youtube.com.

to commit daily to practice the skills we need to feel energetic, clear, centered, and balanced. Many of us are familiar with the cause and effect from caffeine and sugar, poor sleep, booze, and a lousy diet of processed food. We may also know, but not admit to, how it interferes with living and giving. We can presume it adversely affects our patients. We know how much more enthusiastic we feel when we are feeling good. The good news is we always have the option to choose wisely with every choice we are offered.

Maintaining Balance

I offer some *suggestions* (because I know I cannot tell you what to do and no one can tell me what to do either) to aid in feeling more balanced specific to hospice nursing that I learned and earned the hard way. First, I focus on the base needs of eating, drinking, peeing, and stimulation, which segues into the work of spiritual investigation. *Don't start worrying.*

It is difficult when working out in the field to find time to eat in a calm place, and equally important, to pee in a clean place. We cannot function, much less be brilliant with our patients, if our blood sugar is thirty. This is not the place to describe details of a healthy diet, another ongoing issue. I do suggest you eat. I tried not doing this, but it did not work well. Go for enough breakfast to keep your blood sugar up until lunch, lighten up on stimulants and sugars to avoid crashing. Eat enough so that you are not tempted to eat the never-ending flood of goodies at work. Bring good food with you, not Twizzlers. Use a thermos in winter for warm food. Eat lunch slowly, in a lovely, quiet place, even if you are in your car. Stay hydrated. I know it is tempting to stay dry because you do not want to pee often. Make sure you are at least drinking something beyond your coffee. Pee whenever you find a decent potty, and take advantage even if you don't feel the need to go. I have one or two in the county that I rely on. Yes, that's it, but they are beauties. I cannot listen to patients when my bladder is full and all I want is to leave and find that potty. Simple things. I remember an admission when both the social worker and I had to pee even before the admit started, and oh how we suffered. There was no time to go. I vowed not to be in that position again because my attention to the patient and family was sub-par. Poop in the morning at your own home. I would never wish anyone to suffer the nightmare of the sure-to-be-forever reputation a colleague experienced after plugging up a patient's toilet. And you know who you are.

Connect with a colleague. Home-care hospice nursing can be isolating, even lonely, out on the road, and even more so now that we do not have to go to the office as much because we can print from our computers at home. Gone are the weekly team meetings, where twenty staff members gathered to discuss patient care. It was a time to socialize, eat gooey baked goods, and gossip. Without team meetings we have no way to know who is losing or gaining weight, getting married, buried, or delivered unless we make a good effort to find out. Connecting to your people at work can be reenergizing, and it is important to maintain relationships there. I made the mistake of not connecting regularly and felt isolated from my colleagues. I found I was more apt to take comments very seriously and negatively. I felt like an outsider at times. When I did spend time with them I felt better, more connected, and it didn't take that much effort. On the road, you can call your work friends simply to connect, and hopefully you can share some black and horrid humor with them, the catharsis medicinal. Your colleagues will be your most vital support because of their understanding of your work. Hospice nurses report an inability to talk about day-to-day stress of hospice work with family or friends, who naturally cannot grasp fully what we come up against at work or the quantity of daily dramas.

CONSCIOUS BREATHING

One powerful, constantly available method to center yourself is to learn how to breathe consciously. Develop a practice at home so that you can access this skill at any time. There are many to choose from. Please see appendix A, B, and C for ideas.

You can choose to use a breathing technique before you get out of the car to go to a patient's home, again before you knock on his or her door, and when you are feeling some stress in the homes or do not know how to manage a situation. This breath could be a form of prayer that can connect you with your source, whatever form that may take. Breathing with your source can inspire you and calm you down so you can gain insights and find solutions to difficulties in the homes. This calm is a perpetual source of wisdom and available for you at any given moment. It can become a spiritual practice.

PRAYER

Consider building a relationship with a source greater than yourself and speak with it often. Dr. Welch encourages us to "put your worries in the lap of the Divine." *Fear not, Reader!* I am not encouraging anything religious. Divine can be anything greater than yourself, or something you deeply connect with. The divine can be a tree or the woods, an animal you care deeply for, the paints on your artist's palette, the clouds, a saint, the sun, the moon, or the stars. Each person chooses and develops his or her own relationship. I write about prayer because for me praying is energy-and sanity-saving. I know I sound like a billboard outside a church, but I find a fervent call for help is a prayer that I never forget the words to. I have been able to find a solution to difficult symptom management, find invisible veins for a blood draw, bushwhacked through chaotic admissions, and become unstuck in a logjam of questions or concerns using prayer. Prayer supports and sustains me when my esteem dives after making a mistake. I do not have to wait to make a call or go through a menu when praying. Direct answers are available constantly, and they are astronomically better ones than I could ever come up with. "True prayer has no set form.

Just offer your heart-felt gratitude and you will be amply rewarded."[13] A teacher of mine said the other day that "praying is the most powerful thing you can do." And sometimes the answer to my prayer is, "ya better call the office for some help."

If you are not inclined to pray, then kindness seems to be the right thing to do in any situation. There is always a way to be kind. With all the millions of words to choose from to express oneself, there will be a creative way to mix them up to sound genuinely kind and compassionate.

MEDITATION

"Turning within is the sum and substance of all spiritual life."[14]

A renaissance physician said, "Man is ill because he is never still."

OK, so far, we eat, pee, breathe, pray, and next, very importantly, meditate. Start with just one minute, which might be enough to begin to learn to calm the mind. There are many methods to learn to concentrate, which can lead to a meditative state, also included in appendix C.

Meditating might seem impossible at first, and it feels that way often to me still, even after many years of sitting, but it is another one of those on-going, lifelong practices. We commit to meditation or being still for a while every day, and we will benefit mind, body, and soul.

It is important to take time every day to sit in silence, to simply stop and sit. Another influential teacher of mine, Cate Stillman, wrote a book

---

13 Morihei Ueshiba, *The Art of Peace* (Boston, MA: Shambhala, 2010), 41.
14 Swami Paramananda, *Book of Daily Thoughts and Prayers* (Cohasset, MA: Vedanta Center Publishers, 1977), 401.

entitled *Body Thrive*. It is a wonderful resource on how to regain or attain and maintain a balanced state, both physically and emotionally.

To highlight a few of her suggestions, Stillman said:

> To live empowered, you need to clear your mind and digest your experiences. Sitting purposefully in silence, you digest your thoughts, ideas, and experiences. You become available to profound insights and bigger perspectives. You gain access to inner freedom. You tap into a big-time, big-space perspective, which erase the effects of earth stress.[15]

Hospice nurses need the big-space perspective. And we need the quiet, even a small dose daily, of this good medicine.

Hospice nursing is very stressful at times and is becoming more so lately with added technology and a ridiculously increased need for documentation. When I began hospice nursing, we wrote notes with ink, using a cool flip phone with lousy, sporadic service. I had a huge printed map that was like a tarp over the front seat. By the time I left hospice, I had an iPad, GPS, iPhone, and a strong addiction to them all. I was risking my life frequently by driving and talking on the phone. My head was crooked downward from constantly looking down to my iPad during and after work. By the end of a work day, I felt so wired and tired from all the stimulation that my body would recoil from the devices. I felt saturated and drained from hyperconnectivity. And I wasn't fun to be around either, being wired and worried from constantly being connected to work.

Every byte of information we absorb must be digested as if it were food. Both thought and food require space and time to transform to be useful. Overeating and overthinking are forms of overstimulation and stress.

---

15 Cate Stillman, *Body Thrive* (Tetonia, ID: Yogahealer Press, 2015), 179.

Having difficulty digesting a meal is akin to being mentally overstimulated. Our thinking and assimilation become subpar. According to the thousands-year-old medical systems of traditional Chinese medicine and Ayurveda (which hales from India), imbalances are healed by treating with the opposite. This happens in the natural world as well. Light balances dark, heavy balances light, dry balances oily and wet, heat balances cold, and smooth balances rough.

Hyperactivity is balanced with quiet and stillness. Your mind and body crave this, and it is beneficial—no, crucial—to listen to this inner longing.

Overall, I see our society as being more frantic and distracted as our technological devices get smaller and faster, connecting us constantly to people or information sources. Luckily, we have control over how fast we wish to go. If we get ourselves into a frenzy, we are also likely to have our systems crash into torpor and depression from sheer overload. We could instead strive for what Dr. Claudia Welch terms "getting back to neutral," which is a state of peace and equanimity. Getting to a state and feeling of homeostasis is where we can be at ease and most helpful as hospice nurses.

Meditation, diet, and healthy lifestyle are the paths to neutral. "Meditation is our secret weapon, Our savior, and Our Salve. It is a core human need,"[16] Stillman writes.

According to Stillman stress shuts down the frontal lobe, where we do our higher thinking, but keeps the brain stem active. The brain stem is where we react impulsively, or with fear or addictive tendencies. Meditation rechannels blood flow to the frontal lobe from the brain stem so that our responses can change from reactive to receptive, from impulsive to clear and kind, and from compulsive to creative.

---

16 Stillman, *Body Thrive*, 183.

"Meditation builds brain cells, increases gray matter, and allows the brain to slow response to stress, providing better concentration, learning, and memory. This simple practice thickens the part of your brain that makes decisions while shrinking the part of your brain that is active during fight-or-flight response."[17]

Meditation enables your mind to rewire itself, changing the way your brain works, and this expands your potential. As you become aware of old patterns and decide to let them go over time, you free yourself to make better choices and assume a more evolved identity.

Eknath Eswaran said, "When the mind is stilled, ego dissolves." We see the world very differently in meditation; when the senses quiet, so does the mind. As we slow the furious activity of the mind, we can see little spaces between the angry waves, a restful period, and we can work on extending that as our thinking slows down.

"If I can regulate my thinking process, adapt my mental state with serenity, there is no problem that can overwhelm me, no challenge I cannot meet...When we see our negative thoughts during meditation we can sense how quickly they travel and how rapidly they control us. During meditation, as these thoughts slow we realize we can regulate them. As anger slows 'it becomes compassion."[18]

Becoming ruler of your thoughts takes great and steady practice, Eswaran said.

He feels the fruits of meditation are making life more loving, secure, and joyful. In old age we are able to actively contribute to our environment.

---

17 Stillman, *Body Thrive*, 183.
18 "The Training of Attention," Eknath Eswaran, accessed February 2010, www.youtube.com.

To learn several simple meditation techniques, see appendices A, B, and C.

Eat, pee, breathe, pray, meditate, and, oh, try listening to calming music on the radio when you are traveling around during a workday. Save the hard rock for when you are not working to avoid disturbing your nervous system. Getting all revved up on noise is unsettling. Seek calm. Loud and crazy music contrasts your conscious breathing and your quiet being, which is the one you need when with your patients and families.

I have suggested several ways to quiet and balance yourselves. When we are ready to begin to make these small changes, Dr. Robert Svoboda, doctor of Ayurveda and a scholar in Eastern religion, offers these suggestions as a starting place. There are some Sanskrit terms that I needed to leave to quote him verbatim. This is taken from his Web page.

1. Make a commitment to your health.
2. Add and subtract new habits slowly, one at a time.
3. Only once you are stable in a new pattern should you move on to changing or adding another.
4. Pick an auspicious time to begin any new *niyama* (practice). The morning, beginning of the month or year, an auspicious day or time (Jyotisha, or Indian astrology, is helpful for this), or the day after the new moon are all good options. It is also good to fast or purify somehow the day before you begin.
5. Failure happens; don't dwell.
6. Every once in a while, you should break your pattern so that you remember why you are keeping your niyama (practice) in the first place. Don't strive to be perfectly pure—during the Kali Yuga this is not helpful or possible.[19]

---

19 "Dr. Robert Svoboda: On Niyama," Dr. Robert Svoboda, last modified October 2015/ accessed December 2015, www.drsvoboda.com.

EFFECTS OF GOOD SELF-CARE

As we make a commitment to grow, we will discover that people will begin to respond to us in a different way, and we will respond to situations with more clarity and be of more assistance. Once we start to feel the effects of good habits and self-care, we tend to want to build from there. Then we want more. It takes time. Go easy, but go. I had a wonderful teacher who tried to drum into her students' heads that "slowly and slowly" is the way to make a change.

> "If we do not know how to take care of ourselves and to love ourselves, we cannot take care of the people we love. Loving oneself is the foundation for loving another person."[20]

If we are physically and emotionally stable, no matter what the circumstance in the home, we should have a good effect on the household. The families should feel some relief, gain in confidence, and feel less burdened. I felt the most fulfilled in my work when a family member or patient said he or she felt his or her colossal burden was relieved once he or she began hospice care.

Along with being a stable person, we need to be of good character, to have integrity and capacity to stand with people who are under such duress. Sant Ajaib Singh ji Maharaj said, "It is very important for you to have good character, because only then will the healing you are doing be beneficial to the patient. If your character is not good, our treatment will not give any benefit to your patient. But if you have good character, if you are chaste, then it can have a direct effect on the patient and even if you only give

---

20 Thích Nhất Hạnh. *Your True Home: The Everyday Wisdom of Thích Nhất Hạnh: 365 Days of Practical, Powerful Teachings from the Beloved Zen Teacher*, accessed March 2016, www.goodreads.com.

him a little medicine, he can become all right."[21] Applying Dr. Welch's teacher's words to hospice nursing, we see how crucial it is to be centered and clear-sighted with patients and families.

ALCOHOL

I may scare a few of you away right now, but if you feel inclined to drink often please persist to read just a bit more. No one needs to know. I realized drinking affected my patients and families. During my career, I convinced myself I was fine and a good nurse even though many years ago I was imbibing a glass or two every night. Others may feel no effect the next day, but, looking back, I know I was not even moderately focused. I think I provided good enough maintenance care, but I also know I was quick to anger in those days, quick to react to anything. I was supersensitive to any whiff of criticism. I still have an annoying little habit of overreacting, but I know alcohol and feeling badly about myself added to this haste to emote. I know I feel more clear and ready for the job not drinking the night before, and eventually I cut out alcohol nearly completely, never drinking the night before a workday. Alcohol is a depressant, and I was kidding myself that I was not submerged by alcohol's effects. If you like to drink, take a good look at how you feel waking up after no wine and after some wine. Ask yourself honestly which feels better. A preference for feeling very alert and enthusiastic began to replace the sluggishness and blurry mind, slowly and slowly. Preferring this state helped me change my behavior. When I asked my own alcoholic dad, who was not drinking at that moment, how he handled alcohol, he said, "It's better if you don't." He was right. Research your own habits keeping in focus your and your patients' highest good. Think about what your patients deserve.

---

21 Sant Ajaib Singh ji Maharaj (complied by Michael Mayo-Smith), *In Search of the Gracious One: An Account in His Own Words of the Spiritual Search and Discipleship of Sant Ajaib Singh*, (Manchester, NH: Keystone Press, 2009), 209.

Family Reminders

We bring our history and experiences to the job. The complex relationship with our parents and siblings, our angers and fears, can all resurface when we are drawn into the heart and intricacies of another family. We can insidiously be drawn into others' dynamics that mimic those of our family, healthy or not so much. There are triggers and hot spots to be vigilant of. I know I have been drawn to large, chaotic families, preferably with animals (specifically, if you have silly, fat labs and loyal retrievers, many cats, fourteen gerbils, and a house that smells of cedar shavings, I am sold) because that is very familiar to me. I like making people laugh because it meant so much to me to make my dad laugh. That's when I felt valued. Coming from a family of six kids and having an identical twin, I understand sibling jealousy too well. I understand competitive giving and grieving. I understand addiction and alcoholism from my own family. You will see similar personalities in your family and the hospice families you work with. When you feel strong emotion, you may not understand it because some of the reaction is subconscious. Even if you have difficulty verbalizing the emotion, try to discuss it with someone trusted on your team. Maybe all you can say is "I am sad/mad/anxious, and I don't know why." This may help you to separate your history with your family with the case you're working on. It is tricky ground, more like quicksand. If you get in there, remain calm, do not struggle, call for help from your spiritual source. *That again?* Reach for that metaphoric stick, the iPhone, to call your office. I remember all those westerns and Tarzan movies with the bad guys sinking in quicksand, reaching for that stick that was just out of reach. When I picture the hat sitting on top of the quicksand, it still terrifies me.

Getting Involved

There may be a fine line between being a patient's caseworker and one who is overly invested. We can take our work very seriously, and sometimes too much so. You may red flag yourself when you want to be the sole nurse, or the family only wants you as a nurse. You might also feel competitive with the other nurses because you want to be singled out as the best. Maybe you were even told you were the best, and that feels so good. Yet what feels good to the ego isn't always healthy. When you feel yourself reveling in your great work, take note. Being sole proprietor of a case creates a lopsided team. Other clues of dysfunction are when your worry feels neurotic and constant, when you are losing sleep, and losing your sense of humor, and when you request constant updates on your patients. Notice if you become angry or feel threatened when another nurse changes or even slightly alters your plan. Now, why am I familiar with these? It is not something I have read about, or heard from a colleague. Squirm. "Been there. Done that."

Some of us will get very involved because that is who we are. Working intimately with wonderful families draws us right in. It's going to happen. I encourage you to try to notice your attachment and look for insights as to why a particular family draws you in. We all have issues from generations of family baggage, traumas, and our deeper insecurities. A good sense of humor can help you to say, "Oh, there I go again, trying to get my dad to love me, or my mother to listen, or someone to take me seriously for once." Talk to someone if you can about your feelings. Then dilute the care by rallying the force of the team.

I believe if you have a good sounding board at work to talk through your cases and other areas of your life are balanced, you are less likely to become overly involved with your patients and families. To contradict myself, I also find you can be content at home and still become attached. It's a personality thing. I also believe we need genuine feelings of personal worth to be able to do this work over the long haul. Meaningful work can contribute to self-esteem, but it should not be the sole source of your emotional nourishment. When I depended on day-to-day affirmations from others, I was vulnerable to crashing. The sweet, instant high from praise was proportional to my crashing when I felt criticized or neglected. According to the oldest system of healing known as Ayurveda, one definition of health is "one who is situated in the self." The healthy person does not rely on others' opinions to sustain him or her, but is able to feel rooted firmly in belief in him-or herself. I work on this every day.

CHAPTER 4

Healing and Curing

● ● ●

MOST NURSES ARE EDUCATED IN and work in an allopathic setting. The focus in this typical medical setting is on fixing, curing, and alleviating symptoms, all of which are beneficial, but also imply an endpoint. The focus is on the disease. Healing differs from curing in that healing can occur emotionally when disease cannot be cured. A person can be peaceful and have a terminal illness. Due to the more holistic approach in hospice nursing, I have witnessed what appears to be pure grace many times in patients and families. I have more often witnessed the opposite in a hospital setting when the focus is on the physical fix, the person's state of mind ignored.

> "Curing is a focus of an allopathic health care system where a restoring to health, eliminating signs and symptoms of disease and providing remedies for is the goal. Healing, however, is directed toward our wholeness, and may occur without curing. When curing may not be possible, healing is always possible."[22]

Curing often follows a pattern or a predictable path, whereas healing is creative and unpredictable in process and outcome. Death is viewed as a

---

22 Solomon, P. *The X-Factor in Healing.* In *Body, Mind, and Spirit: The Journey Toward Healing and Wholeness,* edited by P. Albright and B. P. Albright (Brattleboro, VT: Stephen Greene Press, 1980), 14.

failure in the modern medical system, whereas in a healing system, death is viewed as a natural process.

> "Techniques are useful, but they are nothing more than a system of exchange for moving energy. None of the technique matters except as a method for transferring that which does matter, which is love in the heart of the healer."[23]

When I think about a person who is dying and healing simultaneously I think of a woman I worked with who was dying from a face and neck cancer. She had colossal faith. Despite weeping tumors, total loss of strength, and being aware death was near, she said she felt well cared for by God. She reported with a smile that she that after she passed away, she would be able to have contact with her children on earth and be able to help them, and even yell at them when necessary. She said, "I am so peaceful. I am ready. I am with God, and I know I am going to be OK." To this woman nothing was lacking in her life or death.

Those who claim to have no faith can also find acceptance about dying and feel complete and healed. One patient, a firm atheist, felt impatient that she was not dying when she wished. She was at ease with death being the absolute end. At ninety-two, she had buried two husbands, said she was tired of being alive, knew her kids would be OK, and just wanted it all to end. She was fearless and firm. Her resolute wish to die, lacking any anger or negativity, was a sign of healing to me. My own atheist father felt his children were his legacy, and this brought him some peace and healing. Another patient, a psychiatrist who was also an atheist, felt love was his religion, and he died very peacefully knowing he had loved well.

While on call one day I received a call from a thirty-six-year-old mother with three children, the youngest only five. She had been very ill with

---

23 Ibid.

breast cancer for five years and said she felt like she had been through hell, like most people with cancer. She had not been admitted to hospice yet, and she wanted to talk. She was extremely ill, and asked me for advice on what to do. She said, "I want to go to the hospital and get IV fluids, so I can go home to be there for my five-year-old's first day of kindergarten. Should I?" We discussed options, and she decided to go to the hospital. Before she left her house, she wrapped her baby in her favorite old sweater. Once there, she became so weak that she could not go home. I spoke to her the next day, and she said to me, "I have suffered so much, and I am so tired. My boat is so small, and the river is so wide. I am ready, Peg, and I am OK." I wrote down her words as she said them, and I told her I would share her story one day. I found it astounding that she reached the point of readiness to leave this life and her children. Her mother called me the next day to tell me that her daughter once again said goodbye and thank you to me, and she told her mom to tell me again that "I am OK." She died that day. Grace.

Most patients in our hospice appear to die at peace. This is the result of their own ideas on closure, how they feel they have lived their lives, and their feelings of self-respect and self-worth. Our guidance in end-of-life care is helpful, but the hard work is done in the hearts and minds of those who recognize they are dying and their families. There is no script to follow. Each of us has our own way to close doors and walk away from this life. Some may do this work in ways we do not recognize. Sometimes I asked a question about something I considered meaningful, and I was given a blank stare in return. This does not mean they are not doing their work. They are just not doing it according to my little list of questions.

The patient who asked me not to return prompted me to ponder the nature of healing. She continued to hope for a miracle until she died. Her Catholic faith was her fortress, the hope for a miracle her ammunition against doubt. This prevented her from discussing death and dying with me, her husband, and her college-age daughter. Though she appeared physically uncomfortable, she accepted minimal amounts of pain medicine, wanting to be alert for that moment of divine intervention. Despite her faith, she seemed to me to suffer unnecessarily. In retrospect, perhaps her image of healing did not fit mine. I am aware Christ declined the wine-soaked cloth before he died. Perhaps she thought her resistance to death was a good example to her family. When I told her the story of the other faithful woman with head and neck tumors dying so beautifully, she barely smiled. She may have resented it. After I told her this story, I never saw her again because I went on vacation. I cannot say whether she was healed or not for we do not decide these things, but to me she appeared to be in spiritual distress. Silly me thought I could get to the root of it. Projecting how I thought I would feel if I were she, or medicating as I thought appropriate, was probably one of my mistakes with her. Offering medicine and discussion of end of life was of no interest to her. She had other forms of healing in mind, which I did not grasp at the time. Maybe healing is not as we imagine. Maybe "at peace" means continuing the fight and being remembered as a soldier. How often do we read in an obit: "succumbed after a valiant fight against cancer." Maybe they want their families to know how much they wanted to live and not leave them, that they did everything possible to stay. In hindsight, I was not perceiving deeply enough to validate her faith.

CHAPTER 5

The Practical Work

● ● ●

PREPARING FOR YOUR WORKDAY

ALL THIS VERBIAGE AND YOU must be aghast that we are not even at the patient's door! Now you see so much needs to happen prior to knocking on a patient or family's door. Well, we are not knocking on the door yet. There is more to consider before you arrive at a patient's home. Buzz sentence, wait for it.

Before you exit your driveway (yes, we are still in the driveway, but at least you are in your car), have at least a vague idea of the patient you will meet. Be prepared. At times I was not. There were occasions when I had no history and physical, just the patient's nutshell version (such as lung disease, dementia, end-stage cardiac disease, cancer). "What's the big picture out there?" I would ask in a hurry over the phone on the way to an admission. Then I would wing it from there. In one home, on not one of my better days, there were two elderly people, both with oxygen, both looking like they might meet hospice criteria, and their names were unisex, like Jean and Alex. I could not tell which one was the patient, so I had to ask leading, sneaky questions to solve the puzzle. Try to get as much history as you can, such as the patient's gender. Another time I was in an assisted-living facility (ALF) and began talking to a woman who appeared frail enough to meet some sort of criteria. Her son arrived, and I mentioned hospice, and he said, "Why is hospice here?" As it turned out, the real hospice patient had been moved to another room and we had not been told. Still, it was my mistake, because if I had more information than a room number I would have known a little sooner.

Find out if the chaplain or social worker will be joining you for the admit. It is so important to have others from the team with you so the family is exposed to the team approach from the start. They play a critical role in trust and rapport building. Sometimes team members are unavailable, and you must do the admission alone, which is not preferred, but it is OK. You build your own confidence this way.

Get good directions to the home. Driving around frantically looking for an address on an unmarked dirt road, with an unmarked house, at night, in the woods, does not set you up for a smooth entrance. Have the family give good directions on the intake form if their home is difficult to reach or see. More than once I did not have good directions (no GPS then) and arrived in a very stressed-out state to do a death pronouncement. I had difficulty connecting right away because I was trying to adjust from screaming at the stupid roads and numberless houses to being supersensitive and connected to someone's monumental loss. Know which direction to go on the highway. I've gone north when I should have gone south more than once. This takes up time and stresses you out. And you shouldn't claim it on your mileage.

Keep the mayhem on your front seat to a minimum. I know what your front seats look like—and your backseats and trunks too. My partner, Roger, named my car the diaper wagon. You create chaos when stuff jettisons all over the car when you slam on your brakes after driving past the house (for the third time) that you have been looking for, for half hour. Documents become wrinkled, and computers don't like being airborne and landing hard on the dashboard (yes, Kate!). "What is that stain on the DNR, Peg?" I have been asked. Coffee cups and computers seem to have the same velocity with hard braking. Shirts and pants can get stained in unfortunate places, so consider drinking clear liquids or wearing dark shirts. Wear a bib. Keeping it simple is another form of self-care.

When you arrive, turn off your music, iPhone, or both for a minute. Take a few precious moments of quiet to ground and center yourself. Breathe and pray. Ask for insight and compassion and to do your best for all involved. Keep this calmness as you walk to the front door. Propelling yourself out of the car without this breath makes you ring the doorbell too many times and your pupils might appear constricted from stress. Constricted pupils make you appear overdosed, or at least frantic, which is unattractive in these settings.

Imagine the person the families you are visiting want to see. Yes, they absolutely expect an angel. This is an awfully lofty expectation that allows for no mistakes or flaws in our characters, and since this is not possible, we must at least attempt to live the golden rule, "Do unto others as we would have others do unto us." We support people as we would want to be supported. I have heard the golden rule reversed as well, "Never do to someone else what you would never want done to you." If I am struggling with the golden rule I will imagine caring for the patient as if he or she were someone I really love. This helps ignite more tenderness and respect.

FINALLY, ON THE THRESHOLD

"Breathing in, I am aware of my body. Breathing out, I smile to my whole body...Breathing in I am aware of my body. Breathing out, I release tension in my body.[24]

If your hospice is sound and solid with kind and patient professionals working in the office (like mine), the reputation may precede your first

---

24 Hanh, *Your True Home*, 145, 266.

visit and the seeds of trust will already have been sown. The doctor's recommendation of the hospice and the first welcoming, friendly phone calls to or from hospice set the tone for their experience. Anticipating their needs at discharge for the home or facility while in the hospital will help create a smooth transition to hospice care and continue to form the foundation for essential trust building.

Hospice team members can remind themselves they are entering the sacred space of someone's home. Consider that you have already been trusted enough just to be invited in. We have been honored with E-Z Passes for quick entry into people's most personal space, to touch them physically and emotionally, occasionally within minutes after entering their homes, at a most vulnerable, painful time. Because of this incredible and nearly automatic response of allowing strangers in, we quicken our deep respect for them even before arrival. They will sense this respect and your integrity when you first meet.

Your peaceful, confident entry continues to support good initial impressions. These signs of respect add sturdy stones to the structure of their hospice experience, for it is from here that we are allowed and privileged to continue building the relationship. The family chooses to listen to our guidance to begin to learn how to care for their loved one. The patient can begin to relax enough to continue his or her work of dying without distraction of worry. When they trust our suggestions for medicine or for bringing in team members or techniques for care, we are setting them up for success, empowering them to cope with this huge event. It is vital that they know we are there for them. Without this trust, the family might feel angry, misguided, confused, anxious, and even abandoned. In other words, they might as well be in a hospital where these emotions are more common.

Ring the doorbell just once or knock two or three times. You may laugh, but if you think about it, knocking more than three times and ringing twice sounds impatient. You want them to feel you have all the time in the world for them. And then some.

When the door opens, smile and make direct eye contact with whoever is there. Offer your hand in a fairly firm handshake, but avoid the wicked firm shake that elicits a wince, which I have been known to cause. Introduce yourself and the team members present. Shine that ID you are presumed to be wearing. There are times when the patient is not ready to accept hospice, but the family is in great need, so hopefully the family lets us know before we arrive if we need to censor ourselves. In the case of needing to censor, I might not shine the ID and say I am a visiting/home-care nurse or adjunct staff there to assist the present caregivers. To me, it is not a big deal if they are not quite ready to accept the philosophy of hospice on admission because eventually, with proper care from the hospice, they realize the help we offer them and their families. Some patients will accept hospice because they know their families need support.

Stepping over the threshold, clean your feet off and ask where they would like you to put your coat and bag versus plopping your stuff down on Grandma's antique. Ask where the family would like you to wash your hands. Sometimes the soap is not obvious, so inquire. Do not start opening cabinets. All these actions imply respect for their space. I will ask, while at the sink washing, how things are going to get a feel how dire the situation might or might not be. This gives me a quick view of how the family is coping and their level of anxiety or exhaustion.

"You can't move fast around people who have been scared by life," James O'Connel said in an NPR interview. Move slowly, exude calm. In the past I was called a bull in a china shop. Now my three favorite words in hospice are *gentle*, *morphine*, and *Ativan*, because of the good effects of each. I love myself when I am gentle, but I had to learn how to go slowly enough to be gentle! Remember that flight attendant. Nurses can be the calm, thus the balm, that patients and families crave.

Speak softly, unless the patient cannot hear you, and then when you ask which is his or her good ear, if the patient has one, speak with a tone he or she can hear.

When you meet the patient, offer your hand again, and if he or she is nonresponsive, gently introduce yourself anyway. If your hands are warm, a soft touch to the patient's hand would be sweet. This shows respect and dignity for the patient and family no matter the state of consciousness of the patient. In hospice, we believe a patient always has some form of awareness until death (and some believe beyond), despite his or her inability to respond.

CHAPTER 6

Beginning an Admission

● ● ●

IDEALLY, YOU HAVE A SOCIAL worker or chaplain with you. Another professional's perspective and support for you and the family is more than helpful.

Admissions can take anywhere from twenty-six minutes to three and a half hours, not including documentation. Just writing about admissions for this book took me six months. During this first visit there is an incredible, but doable, amount to cover even without doing any patient care. More time is needed if the patient needs symptom management. Your first goal is to ensure the patient is comfortable and settled. Some patients are just arriving from the hospital via ambulance and need prompt care. At the very least they are usually tangled in five (not always dry or sweet smelling) sheets and maybe a blanket or two. When the patient is a mess or has pain and anxiety, neither the patient of family members can concentrate on any other tasks other than managing the immediate obvious tasks. Getting settled can be more time-consuming than you predicted for an admission, so it is helpful to go in knowing you don't know how long it will take to complete.

During an admission, the family and patient undoubtedly experience at least some anxiety. They are leaping into unknown territory. They may hold the common belief that hospice is only there for the end, and they are grieving in anticipation. They may also feel relieved to gain support while simultaneously struggling with the knowledge that hospice staff is really in their home. They are worried about their loved one, their families, their schedule, their estranged siblings, you name it, and now they have a whole new gang of people to trust. They are often already beyond exhausted having gotten this far with much less support. And then there is the exploding reality that this beloved person is really going to die, and we are the blaring evidence. The social worker or chaplain will be there to assist and begin to gradually assuage this anxiety.

Attend to basic needs first. If you feel the patient needs immediate symptom management, begin the process of ordering meds and then arrange for medicine to be picked up at the pharmacy or delivered from a remote pharmacy. Ask the office to help if you feel squeezed for time. Ask the team member with you to continue supporting the family while you attend to symptom management. This immediate advocacy continues trust building. If the patient needs immediate care, you may be able to teach the family some simple caregiving techniques, such as a sheet or Depends change, mouth care, or medicine administration. It is my experience that demonstrating care far outweighs mere discussion. Inviting family to participate in caregiving right then and there, if they feel able, improves retention and begins the process of esteem building by showing them they are indeed capable of caregiving. Further instruction can proceed only when the patient is settled and the family less distracted.

Assess who is available for the admission. This may include a spouse, siblings, friends, extended family, or private caregivers. I have overcome my fear of public speaking somewhat by learning how to talk with large numbers of family members. Ask who the health care proxy is if the patient is unable to sign documents.

ADMISSION CONVERSATION

It is helpful to engage in light banter, to find some connection. Being an animal lover, I will zero in on any animal in sight, even if it is a cardinal at the bird feeder. Bonus if the patient has a fat lab. There are usually pictures on walls, and you can ask about grandbabies and kids. The social worker is a pro at this too, and he or she needs to get the patient's history anyway. There is always something to connect on. Don't tell a patient right away that he or she reminds you of your father or mother. Just keep your heart and eyes open.

At times, the patient is too ill or exhausted to be part of the admission conversation and may end up being overstimulated and overwhelmed by the conversation. Sometimes he or she can begin the admission process with the group and then need to rest. So many topics are addressed during an admission, and the patient and family can begin to feel exhausted, so keep your eyes on their body language for fatigue. I have needed to omit less critical topics to get the essential paper signing completed because I notice everyone is becoming pale and glazed from stress.

Gather together where everyone has good eye contact and can hear. You should sit close to the patient, on his or her good-ear side, and as close to his or her eye level as possible. I wear pants or long skirts to work precisely for this reason. I am often kneeling in front of people or alongside of them. Avoid choosing that cute, sexy, short skirt or low-cut shirt to help you avoid an embarrassing moment. You don't want to be worrying, and they don't need the distraction of your wardrobe or its malfunctions.

Describe hospice's holistic philosophy and the team approach as early as possible. Discuss how we attend to the patient and family needs using a team of professionals and discuss their roles. Give some detail of what hospice offers to families, such as medicine management, symptom management, equipment, on-call RNs, and twenty-four-hour assistance. The social worker can describe his or her role and either of you can encourage use of the chaplain, home health aides, and volunteers. Emphasize that hospice strives for a collaborative rather than a hierarchical relationship. Hospice workers are not dictators, police, probation officers, or campaigning for anything other than the patient's peace, comfort, and quality of life.

Roughly 20 percent of hospice patients have some form of dementia, and you will be admitting them at home, or more frequently, in facilities. According to my supervisor, we cannot use the vague diagnosis of dementia since people do not die directly from dementia, but from sequelae such as protein malnutrition or infection. I find these patients require excellent assessment skills because you need to observe almost microscopically to determine changes. Medicare requires measurable data so they can track a decline, therefore you will need to be even more observant for less obvious symptoms of decline. During admission, it is smart to obtain arm circumferences and a weight if possible so that you have a baseline. Over time you can note changes in body mass, appetite, and consciousness. Changes in language or cognition are subtle and sometimes difficult symptoms to track, but tracking them is appreciated by your accreditors and Medicare. Having a good relationship with staff in facilities who care for these people is very helpful, since they have the most intimate relationship with the patients and can provide good data on a day-to-day basis. Begin this vital relationship at admission.

Regardless of where admission takes place, always attempt to make eye contact with patients with dementia. Include them in the process if they are able, and treat them with respect even if you feel they may not hear, respond, or understand you. The family will notice and appreciate the integrity and respect you offer. Speak knowing the patient is listening and understanding on some level even if all he or she senses from you is your warmth.

Atul Gawande, author of *Being Mortal* and a surgeon devoted to quality end-of-life care, describes a significant experience with his terminally ill father's doctor:

> Benzel had a way of looking at people that let them know he was really looking at them. He was several inches taller than my parents, but he made sure to sit at eye level. He turned his seat away

from the computer and planted himself directly in front of them. He did not twitch or fidget or even react when my father talked. He had that mid-westerner's habit of waiting a beat after people have spoken before speaking himself, in order to see if they are really done. Eventually, he steered the conversation back to the central issue. He recognized my father's questions came from fear, so he took the time to answer them, even the annoying ones.[25]

These are qualities and manners hospice nurses could embrace as well.

Speak slowly, but not condescendingly. When my dad was on hospice, he loathed it when people called him honey. I've heard nurses use terms of seeming endearment, like little chicken, my friend, pork chop, lamb chop, sweetie pie, and deary, all of which make me cringe. Neither will you will impress anyone by rapid-fire speech. You are most likely not a CNN newscaster or an auctioneer, so quell a tendency toward fast speech that will turn them off or cause them to tune you out. At the very least, they will be confused with too much information. Slow everything down. I am saying this because I know I have made the mistake of rattling off information to no one's benefit. I might as well not have spoken at all. It is quite possible I was trying to sound like a whippersnapper, smarty-pants nurse by talking fast. Fast does not imply intelligence and efficiency. Aim for clear, kind, succinct, and to the point. The recipients' retention might be better if you stop trying to impress them with your obviously vast knowledge and shoot for clarity.

Some doctors are videotaping office visits as an aid in retention since they find even the most intelligent patients retain very little of the content or instructions. I mention this because retention is poor during hospice visits too, and you will need to repeat most instructions. Writing down

---

25   . Atal Gawande, *Being Mortal* (New York: Metropolitan Books, Henry Holt and Company, LLC, 2014), 198

medicine and staff schedules as much as possible is most helpful. Stress, not stupidity, can cause poor retention.

"The most important thing in life is to establish an unafraid, heartfelt communication with others and it is never more important than with a dying person."[26] Be yourself. Use your sense of humor and your common sense and try to relax. As you relax, so will the patient and family. This helps them communicate, learn and retain. Let them get to know you a bit. This may take some time as everyone has varying levels of ability. Trust needs to be earned. Ask yourself what it takes for you to trust someone.

Heartfelt connection is not always verbal. Silence can be very effective in trust building. One patient told me, "You relax me," and she said it was simply because I was not a big talker, and there was no pressure on her to respond to me. Rinpoche says, "Learn to listen and learn to receive in silence: an open, calm silence that makes the other person feel accepted."[27]

It is important to appear as if you had nothing else in the world to do, even if it is not true. Several people commented to me that my all-the-time-in-the-world demeanor impressed and helped them relax. They said they felt reassured, which buoyed their trust. As soon as a family or patient feels you are preoccupied, the connection changes. They may withhold their questions, feeling it could burden you and your schedule, putting your needs ahead of theirs. If you are concerned about time, then you might have difficulty connecting in a heartfelt way. Your mind is elsewhere, and they feel it. This hurts them. Give yourself enough time for them, and if you feel the admit is taking longer than you expected, excuse yourself and call the office to manage or call your other patients for you. Admissions can be full of surprises, so carve out ample time.

Thích Nhất Hạnh sweetly reminds us to "smile, breathe and go slowly."

---

26 Rinpoche, *The Tibetan Book of Living and Dying*, 174.
27 Rinpoche, *The Tibetan Book of Living and Dying*, 174.

As Ram Dass, a current spiritual leader, said, "We are all just walking each other home," or maybe we are sharing the wheel. I like to think of hospice as the soon-to-be self-driving car. The families and patients are both drivers and passengers. They control as much as they want to, but we, as the programmed vehicle, can drive for them at times, alert for potholes, swerves, and potential obstacles. We have a general understanding of the route to carry them to their destination, so they can concentrate on what is happening in their immediate world and devote themselves to their loved one who needs care. They can sing and cry and write and love without the distraction of worrying about the mechanics. They may then wish to make some decisions, such as how often they would like us to visit, or how sedated they want their loved one to be, and they regain the wheel. Sometimes people want to drive and sometimes to be passengers simultaneously. There is no right or wrong way. The back and forth pulsation of driving and being driven while on hospice can be beautiful, rhythmic, and fluid, akin to the ebbs and flows, giving and receiving, of our natural world.

GOOD QUESTIONS TO ASK

I would like to suggest a few good questions to ask during an admission to serve as a guide. Having your questions and general plan organized in your head helps the admission run smoothly. Without a map, an admission can become confusing, and a nurse could begin to feel that he or she has lost his or her course. Having some handy questions to refer to helps to regain direction. If you need to rein in the conversation, it can be accomplished gently so that everyone's input is respected and appreciated.

Have your itinerary for the hospice admission with you. You could write down a loose guideline of priorities to cover, such as who is caregiving, medicine management, symptom management, paperwork, and DNR. Over time and a thousand admissions, you will develop your own style. No one hospice nurse has the same style, but they can all get the job done well with a little experience. Be patient with yourself. Go out with a few pros to watch how they maneuver about the highways and back roads of an admission.

When the tangents from a family's story seem like a Boston City street map, I might use sentences like: "That's the perfect segue into…" or "Let's continue discussing pain management first and get to the other later," or "We were talking about morphine, so let's concentrate a few more minutes on that." There are many ways to redirect conversation, and you will discover plenty of them. However, please respect what the patient or family was discussing and try not to discourage their ideas or stories. Tell them you appreciate their input, because you do. You want to be alert to their important insights or feelings they may express.

As an opener, I might ask patients and families to tell me a brief history of their disease process. Many of your patients and families have been through the hell of physical pain and medications with challenging side effects as well as mixed messages from the many care providers they have been treated by. Then there is the added depletion of lost hope and staggering loss. Some patients were diagnosed a few weeks prior to their admission and are in an altered state from this traumatic surprise. People's stories can be complex and emotional, and they often feel the need to vent. Hearing their stories is crucial, and your intent listening continues the trust-building process. Your actions and your speech should be trust building. Their information helps you begin to understand their coping methods and some family dynamics, thus helping you begin to formulate a plan for them. This can also make the admission feel overwhelming and time-consuming when there seems to be so much to tackle in a few hours. It is important to make time for it. You will know when to steer the conversation to keep the process moving forward.

Attempt to remain neutral should the patient rant about his or her doctor or previous medical caregivers. Taking either side will escalate emotion and is not helpful to anyone. We do not have full understanding of relationships and dynamics with previous caregivers. Best to remain neutral.

I might ask questions such as:

> "How did you and your doctor decide together to call hospice in today?"

> "What has been going on that helped you make this decision?"

> "What do you know about, or what experience have you had with hospice?"

> "What have the last few months been like?"

> "Any changes in the last few weeks?"

I have found these to be helpful starter questions to warm up the engine.

SELF-DETERMINATION

According to Gawande, people with terminal illness have general concerns: "Avoiding suffering, being with family, having the touch of others, being mentally aware, not becoming a burden to others, and achieving a sense that their life is complete."[28] These are also excellent guidelines for us during an admission.

Let your patients know you are committed to helping them achieve what is most important at the end of their lives. According to Mr. Gawande, other critical questions to ask patients is what they care most about in their

---

28 Gawande, Atul, MD. "Letting Go." *The New Yorker*, August 2, 2010.

50

lives and what having the best day possible would really mean to them. Ask what is most important to your patient and what he or she worries about most. Gawande writes about a woman whose passion was to teach piano. The hospice team set the goal of managing daily difficulties. They ordered commodes, a shower chair, and a bed. They organized help for the bath, and they managed her pain well with various medications. Her anxieties diminished as the challenges came under control. "She was focused on the main chance. She came to a clear view of how she wanted to live the rest of her days. She was going to be home, and she was going to teach."[29] This woman continued to teach until the last few days of life and do what mattered most to her. Our goal as hospice nurses is to know what matters most for these people.

Aside from the self-driving car analogy, emphasize to patients and families that they have control over as much as they want. This seems to come as a tsunami of relief to most people because they have been told what to do medically, usually for years. They may have been hospitalized frequently, and anyone who has been hospitalized understands the feeling of impotency associated with lying in a cold room with an elephant-size gown on waiting and waiting. A patient once said, "To wait is to suffer." Clarify to the family that hospice nurses act as guides/teachers/supplements to the care they already have, that we are not bulldozing our way in to take over and make decisions for them. A hospice nurse's role can change from moment to moment. Sometimes we lead, sometimes we follow. When we deeply perceive, we are sensitive to these fluctuations.

At first patients and families may want hospice on the perimeter of the care they are currently receiving, accepting a nurse visit once a week or even every other week. Gradually we come in more frequently as the need arises or as the family requests. Hospice empowers families and patients to create their own experience of dying.

---

29 Gawande, *Being Mortal*, 248.

As hospice nurses, we can explore and encourage the dying role for patients. Gawande states people want to:

> Share memories, pass on wisdoms and keep-sakes, settle relation-ships, establish their legacies, make peace with God and ensure that those who are left behind will be OK. They want to end their stories on their own terms. This role is, observers argue, among life's most important, for both the dying and those left behind. And if it is, the way we deny people this role, out of obtuseness and neglect, is cause for everlasting shame.[30]

It is painful to consider that people die with so much more to say, unsettled relationships, and unestablished legacies. The social worker and chaplain focus on many of these tasks during their visits, but nurses we can also encourage sharing, establishing, and making peace with others and discussing how the family will cope after the death.

Ira Byock, a renowned doctor and author of *Dying Well* and many other books, has been influential in promoting hospice care in the United States since the 1980s. He encourages caregivers to ask the following:

> How are you feeling inside yourself? Time after time, after a person's physical discomfort had been assessed and the bowels and bladder dealt with, I saw physicians and hospice nurses cut through layers of polite formality and awkwardness with the phrase. I had never heard quite so succinct a way of getting to what seemed to be the heart of the matter, and I was impressed with how consistently the interaction resulted in feelings of deepened understanding and satisfaction for both patients and clinicians.[31]

---

30 Gawande, *Being Mortal*, 249.
31 Ira Byock, MD, *Dying Well: Peace and Possibilities at the End of Life* (New York: Riverhead Books, 1997), 10.

During the admission and each visit to follow, ask the patient and family their perspective on what is going on and what they would imagine optimum quality of life could be. Ask what they hope for day to day and what provokes fear and anxiety. Ask if there are trade-offs they are willing or not willing to make. Mine with your headlamp on for what matters most to this family. Dig for the natural resources that will uplift their experience.

Determine if the patient and family's goal for the patient is to die at home. Some patients might say they would like to go to a facility when they need more care, but they have later admitted to me that their main concern is avoiding burdening their family. Sometimes the family does not feel they have the skills to provide this sort of intimate care. Gently open a dialogue regarding these fears. Encourage people to voice their concerns about someone dying at home. Offering an opportunity to air these fears and teaching practical caregiving skills will boost their confidence. Discuss the strengths of the family and how capable they are to provide the care (in most cases) their loved ones need. Set everyone up for success.

There are times when the patient and family would prefer hospice to continue at home, but the caregivers may, because of age or debility, be unable to provide this. Frequently and understandably, elderly couples want to stay in a home where they have been for decades, and they want to care for each other. The work of caring for a bedbound patient and managing symptoms demands Herculean stamina and is exhausting for even younger people working together. I often say, "This is not a one-man job, and it's a hard two-man job." Begin by finding out who is a potential caregiver. If need be, the social worker can begin the process of finding alternate ways to manage care or begin the painful conversation about the possibility of transferring to a nursing home, assisted living, or even the hospital.

If the situation appears dire, you must begin the process of transfer immediately. It is especially excruciating for the family and patient when the change comes as a rogue tornado. Out of nowhere the wind rushes in and tears you from your old, warm, familiar chair and out of your home—your slippers still under the bed, toothbrush in the rack, a worried cat under the chair, and a bewildered spouse watching helplessly. You are rushed to an unfamiliar facility, into another storm of pandemonium, knowing this is where you will die. I realize I paint a dramatic scene, but this is how it appears for the families when circumstances demand a transfer. You can sense it is very hard to do what is sometimes essential. Even with the best of intentions and with skilled caregivers, not everyone can remain at home. People leave their homes heartbroken, and this is a very painful process for everyone, including you. Know in your heart that sometimes it is the last resort, and you have done everything possible to assist them. Sometimes there is just no other way.

Once they arrive at the facility, it is helpful to have a plan forming with excellent symptom management. Having this relatively under our control alleviates the feelings of helplessness when someone cannot be home.

There are situations when it is reasonable to predict that someone will not die at home, but with support they can remain at home as long as possible. My own mother-in-law was in this situation. At ninety-five, she was unable initially to do much on her own, but with support from family and the hospice team, she remained in her two-room apartment. Either the family or hospice came in three times a day for meals and bathing. She was alert and oriented and wanted to remain where she and her now-deceased husband had lived for many years. She maintained at least fair quality of life watching her favorite cooking shows and Lawrence Welk, maintaining her high level of personal cleanliness, and eating the foods she chose. When she first began hospice, we thought she would decline quickly (what was that rule about having no expectations?) and imagined we could bring her to our home to die when she could no longer manage at home. Her condition plateaued, and our family was ultimately not able to support her in her apartment because our work and home situations could not sustain this. When it became apparent she was more of a chronic patient, we decided with difficulty to place her in a nursing home. She also realized that her needs exceeded what we could provide. With astounding courage and bravery, she walked out her little apartment and did not look back. Later she told me she felt devastated leaving her home.

Families and patients become stronger when they learn ways to cope. When they begin to gain skills in caregiving, scheduling, giving medicine, and changing Depends and sheets, their self-esteem builds. Invite caregivers to participate in as much patient care as possible. Any small act of helping contributes to the caregiver's sense of well-being.

Knowing who will be providing care and having a general plan for down the road is critical to the admission process. As the guide, you need to get a feeling for who will be doing the physical caregiving and the day-to-day care when that becomes necessary. Often this is a difficult topic because most people are surprised and uncomfortable imagining they could truly be bedbound and completely dependent. My mother still believes she will die quickly "like in the movies." Mom feels there is no need to discuss a decline because she won't be doing it. I've stopped reminding her that she has already had one stroke and declined a great deal. I have a feeling many people believe in the movie-star death. From my experience, most of us need a plan, not a director, and the plan begins on admission.

For those fortunate to receive an early referral to hospice, their needs may only be a few hours a day of assistance or —one to two times a week. You can still plant a seed by mentioning that eventually most people require twenty-four-hour care. I will often say, "Should you become too ill or weak, have you thought about what you would like to do and who will be with you?" I often get the look here. They will need someone sturdy enough to be able to care for someone who is bedbound and dependent for all their needs, someone strong enough to turn the patient and change a Depends when the patient can no longer turn him-or herself. Someone needs to be able to do this the twenty-three hours that a nurse or home health aide is not present. I give my line about the "at least two-person job" because of the need for frequent symptom management at the very end of life. I try not to be too dark and gloomy about this, but I do touch on it. Social workers need this information so they can keep in the back of their minds that there is the risk of a transfer to a facility. The nurse needs to document what the plan is, especially if the patient currently lives alone. There needs to be at least a loose plan for care, such as "I plan to have my daughter live with me," or "I plan to go to a facility," or "I will hire privately." You must document something.

A Do-Not-Resuscitate Order (DNR)

We need to bring up the sensitive issue of the DNR during admission as well. I preempt this conversation with: "I need to discuss a sensitive issue. Have you and your doctors discussed the do-not-resuscitate document? Have you heard of comfort measures only?" Maybe the patient already has a DNR, and your job just became a bit easier. Sometimes we start from scratch. I will say, "This is a document that will state your wishes should your heart stop or you stop breathing. It protects you from medical measures that could prolong your life, if that is what you would like to avoid. Without the DNR, you will be taken to the hospital and receive whatever care is necessary to keep you alive, such as intubation, cardiac compressions, intensive-care-unit admission, prolonged hospital stay, and ending in admission to a rehab, which generally lasts many weeks." Most important, offer the generally appealing alternative of staying home and receiving comfort measures to relieve symptoms. Repeat comfort measures protocols. Aligning with people's wishes is where hospice is a great benefit to patients, families, and our crumbling health-care system. Hospice will be called in any of these situations, and we will come to the home to help the patient be as comfortable as possible with medicine and other comfort measures. We make strong efforts to avoid having people go to the hospital when they wish to stay home, avoiding huge amounts of stress and enormous hospital bills. If they choose to sign the DNR, be sure to have the doctor sign promptly because without the paperwork perfectly completed and signed by a doctor, the EMTs, paramedics, doctors, and nurses at a facility cannot honor it. They will do what they need to do to save the patient even if they know it is against the patient's wishes. I have witnesses this very sad scene in the emergency room more than once. It is maddening to witness a code, meaning life-saving measures, being done on a ninety-year old person or anyone else in the end stages of disease.

It is not a priority for a patient to sign a DNR to be on hospice, but it is vitally important to have their wishes documented. Hospice is now required to write a very detailed account of patient wishes, the depth of the discussion, and with whom the discussion took place.

Regularly address the DNR if the patient does not sign right away. This must be done tactfully, or the patient may feel you want him or her to die or that hospice has an agenda. "What's the matter? I am not dying fast enough for ya?" nurses have been asked. A good time to review the DNR is when the patient has declined and a hospitalization would most likely not benefit him or her, which is most of the time. It is very difficult to readdress this when the patient and family are suddenly under duress and need to make a fast decision.

It is not unusual to have a signed DNR, yet when the patient seems to be suffering from respiratory failure, chest pain, or poor pain management, the patient and family will change their minds and wish for treatment. They might decide it is too stressful being home, or they realize they are not ready for comfort measures only and they call 911. The best strategy for this is to try to have a nurse available at the very least to talk to on the phone, or better yet, to make a visit. If the patient goes to the emergency before calling hospice, then the hospice can be very strategic in advocating for the patient by going to the ER. We can be instrumental in helping avoid unnecessary treatment once the patient arrives. It is important to respect the patient's decision to be hospitalized. You might be tempted, like I have been, to wag a finger in his or her face, but this is disrespectful and futile.

I had a patient recently who was ninety-four, and he was a full code for eight months. We readdressed his status a few times, and he was firm about wanting all measures to live. That was fine because the family was on the same page. Suddenly, one day, he had a quick decline in status, and I asked him if he thought going to the hospital was an option. He said, "No, it's too much." His wife and kids were there, and he quickly said, "But if it will be good for everyone else, I will." The family also decided staying home with comfort measures was the right thing to do. It is possible he was thinking of his family when he declined the DNR previously. He always put his wife of seventy years, family, and others first. When there is a split in opinion, rally the team for a family meeting. There may be complex ethical and emotional issues on the table. Attempt to tease apart the fears and hesitations of choosing to resuscitate or not. The issues of what is best for the patient are often rooted in the fears of letting go and control issues among the family members. This can be very complex due to rich and complicated family history. Family members of patients who are not capable of making decisions may prolong the patients' suffering, which makes agreeing on the DNR an important factor in the patient's well-being. If the patient is sound in mind, his or her decision is your focus and no family needs agree with the patient; however, one of our goals is to support the family, so helping them come to an understanding and peace over this death is important.

Many people have the POLST form now, which is very helpful in hospice care. It is a document stating the patient's detailed wishes for medical care at end of life. The patient's doctor counsels him or her and together they sign the document. We are obligated to follow this plan.

Veterans

Another important question during admission is whether the patient is a veteran. Veterans may have different needs that can present with different and increased symptoms at end of life. This could be due to unprocessed witnessed violence, inability to speak to others about their service years, secrets held about their experiences, or perhaps untreated or undiagnosed post-traumatic stress disorder. The social worker and chaplain are a great support to our veterans and make sure they are aware of veteran status after admission if they are not able to attend the admission. There is a great deal we can do as a team to ease their pain and transition.

Maybe not during the admission, but during a quiet visit later, the nurse, social worker, or chaplain can ask gently if the patient was in combat. Your timing will imply your respect for the pain the patient has suffered emotionally or physically. There are vets who have never discussed their experiences. Be conscious of your questions. You could ask something like, "Would you like to talk about your experience in the service?" "Is there someone you would like to talk to about this?" or "Do you feel your feelings about the war affect your quality of life right now?" You can also alert team members who are trained to deal with this very special group of people, but we should be prepared to be present with them if they do wish to talk.

Medication

During the admission, we must attend to the medications. Determine who will be managing the medications or what system they currently have. Ask the family if they prefer nursing to fill and monitor the med box. Often, they are relieved if you take over medicine management. Medicine management gives the nurse a good handle on what is administered and when to reorder medicine. Some folks prefer to maintain control of the medicine and that is their choice, provided you know they are able. You might come across an elderly spouse who feels he or she is able, but your instinct or experience with him or her says otherwise. Promote the idea of relieving him or her of yet another responsibility so he or she can focus on the patient. On admission, go through the scheduled medications, which can be a large handful for breakfast, lunch, and dinner. They may hand you medicine from 2010 or medicine that has been discontinued. Put them in a bag to have family put aside. I have seen cases where every med the patient as ever been on were kept in a dilapidated shoe box. We are not allowed to throw out their medicines. Even meds we order and are delivered belong to the family, so they need to dispose of them. Know your hospice or town policy on this.

If you have comfort meds for the admission, you can prefill and label medicine for the family or teach and demonstrate the methods to fill and administer medicine. You will have to document this and any teaching you do. Teach those who are able how to draw up medicine. This can be an immediate self-esteem builder. They light up and say, "Oh, that's not so hard!" or they say, "How the heck can you read those numbers on the syringes?" It helps them to know that they can help their loved ones be more comfortable (and that it's very easy to be a nurse). It is helpful to bring a medication record so all of you can assess medication effectiveness and keep it organized. This also lifts them up. People love writing down what they have done, because it feels like an accomplishment and proves what they are doing. Of course, any nurse knows this! We just do a little too much of it. It's not that we loathe documenting that much.

Discuss with the family what medicine you feel the hospice will provide and which ones it will not. You may need to call your office to find out the answers to the complicated Parkinson's medications, cardiac meds, latest inhalers, and so forth. Beware. What is covered seems to change daily. I try to give folks a general idea of what will be covered.

Preparing for Typical End-of-Life Symptoms

It is important to anticipate symptoms and teach methods to improve symptoms to reduce anxiety. People are too often admitted to hospice in the late stages of disease with escalating symptoms. We need to let folks know what they can expect. Families have often thanked me for this teaching, for reducing the element of surprise. I sometimes feel as if I land a heavy blow when asked, "How much time?" and I reply an ambiguous "not too much." Often people tell me they appreciated the truth. Preparing the family so that they know their beloved with end-stage cardiac disease could become congested. People with ascites can develop respiratory difficulties. A tumor could bleed or cause increased pain. Patients commonly experience irregular or agonal breathing, confusion, and agitation. Teaching everyone involved what to expect and how to treat symptoms immediately helps everyone cope with these difficult symptoms.

The goal of keeping the patient optimally comfortable not only benefits the patient at the time. It reduces the tremendous stress on the family during and after the death. Families who witness a peaceful death may second-guess themselves less than those who feel the patient did not have a peaceful dying process. Families I have talked to after their family member dies on hospice can torture themselves with self-doubt. They worry they did not medicate enough or medicated too much. They worry they could not stop the secretions. They worry they were not there at the time of death. It could be anything they felt they were slacking on. It is so important as a nurse to let people know how well they are managing the care and what great work they are doing. Caregivers need genuine encouragement and praise before, during, and after the patient's death. Acknowledge caregivers when the patient appears very comfortable, to be breathing easier, and looks clean and well cared for.

Preparing the family for the nearly inevitable confusion and agitation, also known as terminal agitation, is very important. This can be discussed as early as the admission. It becomes frightening to the family when the patient no longer recognizes family members, speaks nonsensically, or is disoriented. Your support is vital here. We cannot know what latent emotion people bring to their deaths. We do not know, and maybe they do not either, what goes on in their sub- or unconscious that needs to be assuaged, laid to rest, or cleansed. This unfinished business may be behind the confusion and agitation, which can sometimes be severe. It is deeply upsetting and exhausting for the caregivers. Be sure to have liberal orders for medicine when your patient is approaching death. On admission, if the patient appears end-stage, seek these quickly.

Morphine

Roxanol, aka, morphine sulfate, is friend, not foe, for most hospice patients and hospice nurses. This is an important topic to delve into during admission whether you feel the patient needs it at the time or not. The family will receive morphine in the comfort pak in the mail the next day, so you want to prepare them. We have received phone calls from frightened family members asking, "What is this stuff doing in my home?" If morphine is there, and you think the patient will be needing it, open it and get that annoying little insert out of the packaging and set the bottle up for people. If they are in a hurry and stressed, opening that bugger will throw them over the edge. They might spill it, too. I have felt this way and spilled morphine.

I will venture to say there is great misperception among the public, and even medical professionals, about this fine friend of hospice nurses and many patients and families. I know other nurses who have come from working in the hospital to work in hospice who are fearful of morphine because the doses seem astronomical to them. A typical dose in the hospital is typically 2mg to 4mg every four hours, and wow, hospice starts at 5mg to 20mg and has no limit! They are terrified they are going to put the patient in respiratory failure. Don't fret. You probably won't. Even if you did cause respiratory failure with narcotics, the patient needed this dose of medicine to be comfortable. We don't give a whopping, huge dose from the start. We titrate the med slowly, increasing as the patient's need for pain medicine increase. Remember in hospice care, comfort first and foremost, and breathing is second.

Ask people what their experience is with morphine, or have them relay stories they have heard. None of them will be good. "Yeah, they gave it to Grandma, and she died with the next breath."

"Our hospice nurse gave my mom the morphine, and she stopped eating and died."

"Hospice comes in and gives morphine so you die. That's what they do."

"Hospice overdosed my son and he died."

"They gave me morphine when I had my appendix out, and I was *out*. Gone!"

Our task is to dispel these myths.

Explain that oral dosing is different from IV in that it is absorbed differently. Reinforce how it is used only as a comfort medicine for symptoms difficult to manage or titrate with pills or patches. Explain the start-low-and-go-slow approach to medicating. It functions as both a pain reliever and a broncho-dilator that really helps people breathe better. I generally throw in that I offer morphine to the oldest and most frail people, and they seem to love it! They dig the euphoria and relief. I have had a few elderly patients on morphine for over a year tell me how much they appreciated it.

Emphasize morphine improves quality of life. It helps patients achieve their personal goals because they are more comfortable. Anyone uncomfortable can only focus on the discomfort. Mention how closely we monitor folks who start morphine. I often give the first dose while present and stay with them a while to support them. I, or another team member, calls the next day to check, and we encourage them to call later if they see anything undesirable. It is also prudent to say, "This is the trial dose. John might need more or less by tomorrow." Reinforce that there is no set dose and that you are flexible and can change it as needed. People like to know there are options. The discussion of morphine is often ongoing because patient needs can change daily.

Now, this is a bit outside the box, but stay with me. What you could do, if it feels right to you, is invite the divine into the morphine. One of my teachers, Dr. Claudia Welch, had a teacher who said, "No medicine works without the presence of God in it," and taught that attention, our directed consciousness, is a link to God, the ocean of consciousness.[32] It is a beautiful idea to me. Use your own experience of what is divine to you. "When we are paying attention, then we are consciously or otherwise bringing an element of awareness and divinity to medicine."[33] What this means to me is that love follows focus. Giving the morphine with love and a feeling of connection to our sense of the divine may be very good medicine.

ADMISSION PAPERWORK

Review services again with everyone and write the schedule for the family, nursing, the aide, social worker, or chaplain. Write down any instructions or medicine schedules you can. Ask about volunteers, and say you will let the volunteer coordinator know their wishes.

Hopefully, either you or the social worker brought the required paperwork with you. There have been times that I would not like to admit I

---

32 Welch, *How the Art of Medicine Makes the Science More Effective*, 95.
33 Ibid.

went paperless. I sign papers toward the end of the admission, after I have already discussed the who's, whys, how's, and what's of hospice care. The paperwork, such as the informed consent, is somewhat of a review. Have the health care proxy (HCP) signed for the patient if they are unable. If you are busy tending to the patient, the social worker can sit with the health care proxy and family to sign the papers. Be sure you have every document that requires a signature. I have lost count of how many times one piece was missing or left in the patient's pile. I am glad you will not be asking a favorite staff member who handles our paperwork how many times I brought incomplete piles of admission paperwork to her. Sometimes I brought the patient's copies instead of the office copies back to her. Poor woman.

Some folks will want to read every single word of each document, which will feel interminably long to you and you will want to scream. You just need to breathe and allow this to happen, even if you know they have dementia and are not retaining anything. Remain calm. Give space. Use this time to reconnect with your breath or another family member.

Give the hospice phone numbers to the family, one for the refrigerator and some for the phones. Write down an alternate number in case the phones go down at your hospice. It is terribly frustrating and a real trust breaker when this happens and a family cannot get through when they are in a crisis.

Vital Signs

We only want to use vital signs to improve comfort, not increase stress. I decide whether to take vitals case by case. Sometimes the patient or family wants to hear the numbers or may expect you to because it is expected that nurses to do this. In my opinion vital signs can cause more stress because the family puts great emphasis on the readings when vital signs, at a certain point in a patient's decline, may have little meaning. I have encountered patients with normal blood pressure who die quickly and those with very low pressure who linger. Some people with a respiratory rate of six per hour live for days, and some in rapid atrial fibrillation live for weeks (generally life-threatening). I have had patients who had perfect blood pressures, oxygen saturation, heart rates, and were alert until the last few moments of life. Because these examples have happened so frequently, I do not put much stock in vital signs.

On admission, I take an initial set for baseline readings and then at least once a week if they are on antihypertensives, cardiac medicine, or diuretics. Weekly weights are helpful for those with renal, liver, or cardiac failure because they might benefit from comfort meds such as diuretics. If these patients are bedbound, I just do my best to assess fluid levels. Those patients who are being audited after slowly declining (never use those two words in your documentation) or plateauing to a relatively stable state need vital signs as evidence of decline, especially their weight, and/or arm circumference, which are documented with vital signs. Ask for your hospice's policy on this.

A nurse can see and understand without her stethoscope, blood pressure cuff, and finger probe. Your visual assessment of respiratory rate and audible breath sounds alerts you to how well someone is oxygenated, and his or her pallor and skin temperature are indicators of blood pressure. When a patient is asymptomatic, I avoid aggressively trying to improve vital signs. I have been pleased how often position changes alone help people and improve their vital signs. Simply dangling a patient at the bedside can ease breathing, joint or muscle discomforts, and lift spirits. Turning to a different side, using pillows brilliantly, easing up on sodium or fluids, opening the windows, or using a fan nearby can alleviate symptoms remarkably. Increasing the per liter flow of oxygen may seem minor, but is very helpful. A low dose of narcotic or sedative can sometimes improve vital signs if alternate methods do not produce desired effects.

WHEN TO LEAVE THE HOME

Not yours, you silly. After an hour or so into the admission process, check in with everyone and note fatigue levels, especially that of the patient. When the admission is happening in the patient's room and the patient appears exhausted or overwhelmed, I will ask if it is OK if we change location and sit in the living room so the patient can rest. Check in with the family as well, who may be equally overwhelmed. The family is probably starting the admission process exhausted. When you see they no longer seem to concentrate or appear saturated, or seem anxious to get up, you should close the admission process. Once questions are all answered for at least this day, the patient is comfortable, and meds understood, then it is OK to leave. Reaffirm the next visit and commit to a call the next day. Make sure they are comfortable and feel at least a little confident in their caregiving.

Calling a newly admitted patient the next day is imperative for several reasons. You continue to form the foundation for good rapport and trust. You need to know how efficient the med regimen is. And you need to check on symptom management in general. However, trust is the most important reason to call. Make sure they received their new meds if ordered and follow up with the pharmacy if they have not. Because of the obvious stress and distractions during an admission, much information was not retained or even heard. The follow-up call is another way to ask if there are questions and to fill in gaps. Ask if there are any other concerns. Ask how everyone is sleeping and coping. Inquire if the family is satisfied with how the patient appears today. Ask if they would like a nurse to visit. Most folks new to hospice will have questions because the experience is full of firsts and the learning curve straight up.

There, see? That admission only took fourteen hours.

CHAPTER 7

Ongoing Work Post-Admission

● ● ●

GOALS AND HOPE

"HOPE IS IMPORTANT BECAUSE IT can make the present moment less difficult to bear. If we believe that tomorrow will be better, we can bear a hardship today."[34]

Experiencing even the slightest feeling of hope lightens the burden of the terminally ill. In-depth discussions of hope can be addressed by the chaplain or social worker, but nurses benefit from understanding the patients' and families' need to feel hope. Hope can be experienced as long term, but also day to day and even hour to hour. One can hope to go to Aruba next month, hope to be alive for a grandbaby's birth, or hope to be pain free or breathe better today. One can hope to eat his or her mom's apple pie today or sip a Fribble from the DQ. Hope, big or little, I imagine, feels the same.

Yet there are pitfalls to avoid concerning hope. In the words of Dr. Welch, "Thrusting hope at someone like it's a lollipop may demonstrate ignorance of how the person is feeling or of what their condition really is."[35]

---

34 *Peace Is Every Step: The Path of Mindfulness in Everyday Life*, Thích Nhất Hạnh, Goodreads, accessed 2016.
35 Welch, *How the Art of Medicine Makes the Science More Effective*, 131.

I had a good friend who was a patient in our hospice. She held tenaciously to the goal of wanting to see her son graduate from college. She could support him emotionally and raise her own spirits through her final days and his senior year by holding this dream close to her heart. Despite profound weakness, she never lost hope that she would be able to go to the ceremony, even up until the last few weeks of her life. I feel this made the dying process more bearable for her. Her hope to see her son graduate and to be there for her other two children (her youngest only twelve) was vital for her last few months of life. She was unable to attend the graduation, but the family was creative and filmed the graduation for her, so she saw him throw his cap and flip his tassel, albeit from her bed. What she hoped for manifested of its own accord because everyone left it wide open to opportunity. No one ever dissuaded her from going. She needed to make her own decision. Our role is to support, no matter what we feel might not be feasible. Undermining someone's goal chips away at his or her life force and sense of freedom. There is always a way to support someone. Dr. Claudia Welch says, "I'm not sure that there is a difference between hope and false hope. There may just be hope. And hope is a far better place to live than hopelessness."[36]

OPTIMISM

Optimism can be contagious, but so can pessimism. We must never cause someone to feel demoralized. We try to buoy patient and family spirits by focusing on the healing we see. We can support the emotional or physical comfort our patients describe to us. I try to avoid words that measure since quantities and qualities in hospice are short-lived. Saying something like, "You are eating so well today" or "It's great you could get to the bathroom by yourself" may sound supportive in the moment, but the day will invariably come when the patient loses his or her appetite or

---

36 Ibid., 129.

becomes unable to walk, and this may cause the patient to feel discouraged. Even saying, "You look great today!" may come cheerfully from your mouth, but the patient could feel horribly sick in the next hour, or maybe he or she feels like hell today and thinks you are not perceptive enough to see it. I try to avoid the words *good* and *bad*. Our casual opinions carry weight. Try to avoid superficial statements that leave you both feeling empty or even dishonest. I loathe it when I hear others say of a patient dying of dementia, "Oh, I just love her. She is so cute." It sounds dishonest and vacant. Your buoyancy may fall flat. I ask the patient what the day is like for him or her, or how it feels to sit in the sun, eat breakfast, drink the protein smoothie, or be with the grandchildren. The patient gives me the information I need.

"Optimism is neither a practice of denial, nor is it a reflection of naivete. It is choosing to perceive and attend to the positive aspects of a situation."[37] When we are calm and open, we can be inspired to see subtle, positive aspects.

Nurses can promote hope and add to quality of life by thinking outside the box. I had a very sick yet vibrant patient in her forties who desperately wanted to swim. She had a subcutaneous pump for pain management. She was weak but ambulatory and very eager. She had no open wounds. Soon enough we spied the friendly neighbor's pool. With neighbors cheering and off the time clock, we took her in a wheelchair to the pool, bolused her with medicine, removed the tubing extension, and in she went. The joy of seeing her face and to see her swim I will never forget. She was thoroughly thrilled, and it boosted her confidence as well. We did this twice before she died. After each dip she said it was well worth it. Knowing the effects of these small acts would bring peace of mind to patients and caregivers, I have also walked dogs, shoveled snow for dogs to play or when patients worried about visitors coming

---

37 Welch, *How the Art of Medicine Makes the Science More Effective*, 12.

up their walks, cooked small meals regularly for those who lived alone, watered gardens for the gardeners, filled bird feeders in snowstorms for the bird lovers, and washed some dishes for a distraught, sick mother. Being creative with care is uplifting for all. Options can breed a feeling of hope.

Being unsure of their capabilities and believing you know the answer, patients and family members may ask whether you feel they are able to fulfill lifetime or day-to-day dreams on their bucket lists. They may want to go to Florida one more time, NYC for a few days, make one more killing at the casino, dine at their favorite restaurant, drink a very old scotch, or fulfill any number of dreams. There will be as many dreams as there are people. I do not discourage them, whether it seems preposterous to me or not. My opinion sprouts from a mustard-seed-size amount of information. People need to continue to unfold their lives. So we start to build their plan together by discussing their current energy levels, project how they might feel wherever they go, how they will manage exhaustion or symptoms while away, and what the short-and long-term goals are for this experience. Help them consider options if they run out of energy, need to rest, or become overwhelmed. Most likely, they will be exhausted by the effort, but for some it will be well worth it. Instead of trampling on their hopes, support their ideas by giving them all the information they need to make their own decision. Allow them the space and time to do their own research on themselves. Discussing their hopes and dreams during an admission works well if people feel they have a fair stretch ahead of them and feel energetic.

Our role is to support whatever is meaningful for the patients and families. Years ago, I read a patient's remark that has stayed with me since. Even if you are unable to do anything outwardly, "at least look like you are trying." There is most always *something* we can do to relieve discomfort. Maybe our trying looks like simply and peacefully sitting at the bedside. Sometimes this is all that is needed.

It is said that nature abhors a vacuum, and hope does too. Dr. Welch said, "Even if the ultimate outcome is death, we can take the time to perceive the patient and reality as fully as possible and as well as we can, and together, wait patiently to discover the hope that is real. When we don't go frantically searching for hope, and we simply wait for it, something real and tangible may arrive to represent hope."[38]

---

38 Welch, *How the Art of Medicine Makes the Science More Effective*, 131.

CHAPTER 8

Control

• • •

HOME

ISSUES OF CONTROL CAN CROP up in any area of hospice care. Conscious patients need to have a say in who comes and goes in their homes, what medications they want, how much they wish to communicate, when to sleep, what to eat, even how safe they want to feel. As patients lose control of everything they have earned, known, owned, and begotten, nurses can provide creative alternatives in these areas. For instance, a nurse can assure the patient that he or she has control over the amount of medicine he or she wishes to receive. A nurse can help the patient choose a lower dose of medicine that may increase symptoms but allow for added awareness, or a higher dose with potential for less awareness. I will ask people who are overwhelmed by their prolonged dying process if they wish to sleep more, and I might encourage them to take the ordered dose of sedative or seek an increase in the dose. I offer Lifeline to the more independent people, even though often I hear a defiant no to this question. We can offer home health aides and other team members. Patients might deny needing more services, but they must be given options. Whenever possible, the patient makes the decision, and if he or she cannot, the health care proxy and family will. The patient does not have to have a bath, get dressed, eat, or follow your (or anyone else's) agenda. Trying to persuade the patient to do anything other than what he or she wants violates the patient's freedom.

The patient and family need to feel in control of their home. Once a patient is admitted to hospice, the home can be flooded by visitors who suddenly feel the need to see the patient. Illness and death can be attractive to some family and friends who want to be involved in a drama, who might need attention themselves, or feel guilt over past experiences with the family or patient. Recommend the family advocate for their loved one by being gatekeepers to the visitors and callers. This control comes as a surprise and relief to patients and families. Kindhearted people feel awkward saying no. Remind them they can limit visits to even a few minutes. Patients have told me, "I did not have the heart to ask them to leave. I don't want them to feel bad," but sadly, the patient feels more drained following the visit. Many people will come to say goodbye, which further depletes the patient. When I query further, often the patient did not feel the need to see or say goodbye to some of these people. Ask the patient who he or she needs and wants to see and have the family witness this request and attempt to uphold it.

Encourage family to notice visitors who add to their experience versus those who require energy to have around. Encourage an attempt to filter, or at least curtail, those who require energy to a short visit. At the end of life, even the most beloved family members' visits can cause the patient to feel exhausted. I remind families that patients are so profoundly fatigued by the smallest efforts that they are unable to respond in their usual way.

As life ebbs, I notice most patients will seek comfort in a peaceful, small, familiar, nest-like space. They will probably desire only their core caregivers to be present, and the caregivers, I find, want this lower stimulation environment as well. During this slowing down and letting go process, they crave quiet. They have no energy for conversation. Noncore family and friends, now nudged to the perimeter of the caregiving, continue to want to participate, and luckily there are ample opportunities to support in other ways by doing housework, shopping, taking or making phone calls, and other loving maintenance activities.

The patient may show less interest in others, and everything external for that matter, other than having comfort needs met. This detachment can be disconcerting for some more distant family members. To me, this is not for lack of love, but rather a sign of the patient's letting go of the material forms and relationships related to this world. There may no longer be anything to say once the enormous energy needed for saying goodbyes are complete. The patient can no longer muster the energy to continue to reconnect over and over. He or she is pulled inward. I see it as a gentle releasing and withdrawal from the world of form or a transitioning to wherever it is we go.

APPETITE

A patient's appetite can become a control issue. His or her appetite tends to become a focal point for close and extended family members, friends, and even neighbors and can be a vehicle for them all to attempt to exert some control. The daily intake becomes the measure of whether the patient is declining or progressing. Many of us instinctively feel the drive to feed someone who is ill, to nourish the person and help him or her recover. Inevitably, patients lose their appetite, and it is at this pivotal time when families feel even more powerless. A patient's waning appetite is a painful turning point in the patient's illness and the families growing awareness of death. Your role is to support both family and patient. The patient needs you to advocate for his or her not eating, and the family needs to be taught about the natural flow in the dying process. They must be encouraged to notice the patient suffers when he or she eats due to the inability of his or her digestive system to cope with nourishment. Emphasize the patient is not hungry, therefore, not starving to death. Starving implies hunger and longing. Remind them that they are not withholding food and causing the starvation—the patient would eat if he or she wished.

This becomes more complex when tube feedings are involved, since the caregivers control the volume and rate of the feedings. It is important to have conversations early in the hospice process regarding the pros and cons of a tube feed, signs and symptoms regarding changing tolerance to food, what to do, and how it will feel to eventually turn off the feeding.

Sometimes, to please and appease, patients force themselves to eat even if they experience no desire for food and even discomfort when eating. Patients often lose their sense of taste prior to losing their appetite, and food is simply not enjoyable. Initially, they may feel indifferent toward food and then it can become something they dread. Eventually, the patient will be unable to maintain attempts to please the family because food will cause such discomfort, or he or she becomes too disabled to eat or swallow.

You can support the family with education around end-of-life care and offer options. I ask the patient in the presence of others if he or she is hungry. If the patient says no, we discuss what may be comforting to do instead, such as popsicles, ice chips, or sips only of certain fluids. I ask what the patient craves, and the answer may be nothing. I reassure the patient this is OK and expected. I've had patients say they wanted some scotch or a beer, and just having the option of having a sip or small taste of food was all they decided they needed.

It is helpful to avoid praising or criticizing someone for eating or not eating (or for anything for that matter). There is no right or wrong, good or bad, and nothing to control. They are doing what they are capable of that moment. It may feel patronizing to the patient when you praise him or her for eating all his or her scrambled eggs or drinking his or her milk. Tomorrow he or she might not care one whit about eggs, and he or she may feel badly that he or she is not being a good patient or pleasing others.

Once the patient stops eating entirely, the family's feeling of powerlessness may prevail. Family members need to be able to contribute, to express their love, and to feel included. Teach and encourage bedside tasks, such as medicating, providing mouth care, turning, cleaning, dressing, hair brushing, and applying lotion. Offering methods to give personal care can relieve the feelings of helplessness. I feel this teaching is critical for the family's well-being following the death.

Continuing the discussion of control, some folks may feel overwhelmed by too many choices. Nietzsche said, "The awesome gift of freedom causes despair." Sometimes the patient and family are too exhausted to cope with more decisions. There came a day when my good friend, who had been a hospice nurse and then hospice patient, asked that I and her team tell her what to do. She half meant it, but there were times she did not wish to be making decisions after having gone through seventy-something doses of chemotherapy and several surgeries. She trusted us. She was depleted and wanted help at times. Being a nurse and very intelligent, she managed her dying process gracefully, but once in a while she wanted at least the option of having someone else in authority.

Timing

I imagine many people feel this sort decision fatigue. Supermarkets use decision fatigue as a strategy to get us to spend more when we are vulnerable. After scouring the aisles and making possibly hundreds of decisions about drinks, bread, milk, cereal, and eggs, our last stop is the register. There we find even more nonessentials like little lighters, candy, Rolaids, and very enlightening/frightening magazines. Those in marketing and advertising are aware customers have no resources left to deliberate at this point. With our fortitude tossed way back in the produce section, sugar and junk cravings can easily overwhelm us, and we spend. After traveling leagues through their illnesses, patients are in a similar state of vulnerability, so some patients look to us to help them make a decision. Continue to educate pros and cons of both sides of what the patient is trying to decide and collaborate with the patient and his or her family. If the decisions are too difficult for the patient to make, suggest doing nothing for now. Just sit with it. Time may open some space for the answer to reveal itself. I am a great believer in this approach.

Another patient of mine, a judge, developed an infection in his last few weeks of life. He deliberated on whether to take an antibiotic because he was end-stage but still mentally lively. He decided to get the medicine from the pharmacy but then opted not to use it. He needed to know there was no good or bad decision and that the decision was his. Either way he would be kept as comfortable as possible. His *ability* to choose and control his outcome, his wife later told me, was the optimum support he needed at that moment. She wrote me a note following his death and said, "I love your drive to illuminate the importance of helping people to live the way they want to at the end of their lives."

Often families choose to treat infection to control the dying process and buy more time. It may also be difficult for them to consider saying to themselves or others that their loved one died of a bladder infection or pneumonia. Treatment might buy a little time. It might relieve an uncomfortable symptom. But here's the rub. The patient will die of something else, and maybe something more distressing. In my opinion, when we are very old or very sick, we are given opportunities to die, and maybe we should consider taking that chance to go. Why wait for cancer to progress, heart disease to further debilitate, a death from respiratory failure, or the malnutrition of end-stage dementia to take control of the dying process? Remember the adage "Pneumonia is an old man/woman's best friend"? If symptoms are manageable, why not let patients take the door that is opening right now? Families might not feel ready for the death, but watching the person die in more misery later will be more tortuous and stressful for everyone.

SAFETY

Safety is a fiery issue and falls right in there with control. The agencies who accredit hospices these days seem indifferent to the time required to document our attempts to keep patients safe. At times our attempts seem futile. The hospice team sets up conditions to improve safety, but we have no control over patient safety. Because our focus is on patient and family independence and dignity, we sometimes see them in unsafe situations. *OK, we often do.* We say we fear for their safety as if falling was the worst thing that could befall them, but in my mind, the worst that could happen is that we trap them in a wheelchair and put more controls on their every movement. (Please God, don't let anyone do that to me!) Yes, sometimes people fall and hurt themselves, break something, end up in a hospital, but they are going to do that anyway, regardless of whether there are care-givers present or not. I have seen patients fall smack-dab in front of me, because once they are going down, unless you are under their arms, you will have less than a second to get to them. You can try your best to make them safe, but I can tell you, once you walk out that door, the joke is on you. I saw a man carrying his walker in the air out in front of him. I've seen many walkers in the middle of the living room. I had a man, an old lawyer, who firmly refused to have anyone, even his kids, stay with him. We all knew he drank beer and whiskey at night and was weak, confused, and unsteady. He had already fallen many times and tried to hide the skin tears and bruises. This man had been a lawyer, and he would smile at my lame recommendations and say, "I will take that under advisement." He rendered me nearly powerless, which is good. I documented my efforts to ensure safety, but it was done with humor, knowing he was going to do whatever he wanted. The patient's family agreed that their dad needed to live by his own rules. Epilogue to the story; he died at home because his decline occurred very quickly. One day he was walking, the next day he was too weak to do so, and he died within a few days with his children there. His wish was granted.

Mr. H., a patient in his eighties, smart, six-foot tall, distinguished man, was having a hard time adjusting to his very recent diagnosis of melanoma with brain metastasis and was in disbelief at the speed of his decline. He was barely walking because of his weakness caused by advancing disease. His overwhelming weakness and near inability to walk bewildered him, but he wanted desperately to walk downstairs to his garage to see a fast and classy car he recently purchased. I doubted he could make it down the stairs, but I said nothing. Instead, I helped him stand. He stood and took a few steps and realized, grief stricken, that he could not possibly make it. Being able to draw his own conclusion about his strength helped him swallow the disheartening blow that he could no longer walk any distance. My assuming the role of a parent would have been disrespectful. Even when you predict patients could fall, all you can do is show them what could make their lives easier and safer and let them be. Give them phone numbers for the nonemergent fire department line. I have had families develop a close and entertaining relationship with the local fire department. Order Lifeline if you can. Alert and prepare the family of the probability of falls, and create a system for help when it occurs.

I had another patient who refused to wait for her home health aide to arrive to take a shower. She was adamant about taking a shower alone, so she did, despite the Parkinson's disease that severely disabled her. I tried to schedule visits at shower time, but she would always just be drying off and smiling when I arrived. Another patient was falling constantly and her exasperated caregivers could not support her weight any longer. I told her she had to stay in bed. (I did? Yes, in my earlier years.) She said to me, "I will not be bedridden the rest of my life. I will get stronger." All night she did leg lifts and, by joe, she got out of bed sans diff the next morning. I ate crow for breakfast.

Returning to a theme, relinquish your control as much as possible by giving them the dignity of choice. Chart your instruction, and let it go. You will look good on paper, and sometimes that is the best you can do. At least the audit will look good.

Patients with dementia who have some awareness of their surroundings can still be offered simple ways to maintain feelings of control. Dementia care is a very large topic, and I discuss it briefly later.

Dangers such as fire risk, violence, and neglect must be attended to, reported, and documented. I have had a few confused patients who wanted to cook, and a blind man even used the stovetop as a heating source. If you feel a patient is not capable of cooking or using a microwave, seek alternatives, such as family providing meals or Meals on Wheels. There are gadgets available to lock the stove controls or burner knobs can be removed. When there is potential for flames near oxygen, you must teach and remind. Some people who smoke have such difficulty letting go of their cigarettes that the risk feels worth it to them. I had a patient recently in this bind. I reminded him that we would not be able to get him or his paralyzed wife out of the apartment in time to save them and that he was putting the whole building at risk for injury. I encouraged everyone to smoke outside. Yes, even in the winter. If you feel unsafe, let the family know.

Violence and neglect must be dealt with immediately. Notify MSW and your supervisors. Document every detail. If you feel physically unsafe, call the police right from the home. Ask your hospice for their policies on this. Bring another team member with you if you are uncomfortable emotionally, but feel safe physically.

ARGUING

Arguing with patients or families may be to attempt to control them. Arguing may also reveal our own fear of being wrong, of not getting our way, or not being able to control a situation. It is tempting to sway patients and families to believe as we do. For example, perhaps you do not believe the patient should go to the hospital for IV fluids, or any treatment, or you feel another patient should not have any more tube feedings. Maybe you think a patient should have a DNR, or you feel the patient should have more medication. I say no shoulding on people. Our role is to provide information—about what the hospital stay would entail, how they might benefit or not from IV fluids, tube feeding, a hospitalization, or not having a DNR. Allow the decision to come from the patients if they are able, or the family, so they can feel a sense of control and have mastery over destiny. They need to feel good about their decisions so that in the future there is less chance for damaging self-doubt. Arguing also implies you think you know best, which implies your belief in your superiority. Wanting to be right also implies you are invested in the outcome of the argument. The only outcome nurses *should* desire is for the patients and families to feel comfortable with their decisions.

Most patients want and need to retain as much control over their lives as possible. Consider the losses they are adjusting to. It is helpful and realistic to remind ourselves that one day we will also lose it all; we'll have to let go of every possession, every person, and every personal identity marker, such as lawyer, writer, nurse, mother, machinist, runner, beautiful (not), a superior athlete, and so on. We lose all physical strength and sometimes even our personalities. Therefore, our job is to help patients and families maintain whatever there is to control and nurture a sense of integrity and dignity. Let people do as they wish within reason. Nurses are not the police. No matter what your opinion, let the patients do their own research and reach their own conclusions. Eventually, everyone discovers what they can and cannot do.

MEDICATION

Many hospice nurses have a story or two of how they, families, patients, or staff in facilities has occasionally given too much, or more commonly, too little comfort medication. Fear of harming, fear of oversedating, lack of education, and wrong medicine may be the underlying issues for under and overmedicating. It is important to educate ourselves and others and advocate for comfort in line with the patients' wishes.

Patients may be over-or under rmedicated if the drug is not the correct one for them. A dose of a wrong drug will not alleviate symptoms and may have the opposite effect. For example, we may increase a dose of morphine if respiratory distress has not been relieved and even continue to increase it when a patient does not respond. Then we realize the patient really needed 120mg of lasix to relieve their congestive heart failure. The patient may then be overmedicated. Some patients have no tolerance for certain meds and any amount may cause them to feel overmedicated. Others who have been on medicines for a long period of time may have developed a tolerance and require large amounts of medicine. If the hospice does not know this patient well, he or she may be prescribed too low a dose at first.

The tough process of letting go is evident as patients and families enrolled in hospice learn the process of medicating. Families who struggle the most with detaching might have difficulty medicating their loved ones optimally since they may prefer the patients as alert and engaged as possible. They may have unfinished business with their sick loved ones. They may not be able to bear anticipating their loss. If you notice a patient is under medicated, you must bring this to the family's attention. I might say gently, "I see John is frowning, and his brow is more deeply furrowed today. I did not see this yesterday. I see he is squirming more today and is moaning at times. What do you notice about John today?" Then I might say, "To me, John appears to be in some pain, evidenced by the furrowed brow and the restlessness. These are the nonverbal cues that patients give us when they cannot describe discomfort for themselves. Would you consider a trial of giving this med more frequently, with a slight adjustment to the previous dose, and see if we can get him to relax?" Offer them the time to talk through their fears with medication and narcotics. Instruct the family that their person does not appear overmedicated since he or she can open his or her eyes, is alert, the pupils are not pinpoint, yet he or she still seems uncomfortable, even while sleeping. Because hospice nurses promote peace and comfort, we are responsible for addressing patients' pain, especially when patients are unable to communicate. Educate the family on subtle signs of discomfort, and focus on helping the family talk about pain management.

Caregivers sometimes feel reluctant to have the responsibility of administering medication, especially narcotics. Education, practice, and reassurance are the antidotes to this fear. Families may undermedicate their loved ones because of fears of overmedicating them and killing them. I have heard caregivers say they do not want to be the last person to give a narcotic because they feel a direct connection between the last dose and last breath. Emphasize that the medication you, or they, are giving is only given for comfort and not to hasten death, which of course is not allowed in most states. If the person dies soon after being medicated, it is probably not related to the medication, but rather this was the right time for this person to die. Caregivers may also fear they caused their sick loved ones to be so medicated that they could not express themselves fully in their last days or hours. It may be true that the patient needed more medicine at the very end of life, but remind them that withholding the medicine may have heightened the patient's discomfort in their remaining time. Normally, most people have a period of a week or more of being nonresponsive. The nurse can help the caregivers know they helped the patient ultimately be more comfortable and die in peace, fulfilling the goals that were established on admission. Obtaining the desired results of the patients being calm and pain free is an ongoing process for some patients and families because they need to be able to trust the medicine is not going to have undesirable effects.

It is very important to have the family feel at ease with the amount of medication they are administering. If the patient does not die well in their eyes, either because the family feels they were overdosed or uncomfortable, their doubts might cause them to have more difficulty with their grief.

There are some categories of patients and families we find the case of over-and undermedicating are veterans, patients with younger children, those with a history of addiction, and those who have a generally stoic view of pain.

Veterans may avoid mind-altering medication. Veterans have said to me, "My buddies bore the pain, so I will too," "I don't want morphine because they used it to help my friends die on the field," or "I survived, so I can at least bear this pain since they gave their lives." One said, "It feels like defeat" (to take meds). For these veterans, ongoing support could be in the form of statements like, "This med will alleviate some of the pain, so you can enjoy your family more. The doses we give are strictly for pain management, like Tylenol, and in proper dose add to quality of life"; "Addiction is not generally an issue in hospice, but to reassure you, I do not notice you asking for the med unless you are uncomfortable. An addict would continually seek the drug"; or "Observing suffering was so difficult during your term of service, and now you have an opportunity to protect your family from seeing you suffer." Remind him or her that suffering can distract from the preciousness of the moment and the quality of time he or she has left to live.

On the flip side, I had a vet who admitted to a history of alcoholism and drug addiction and had been clean long before he came on to hospice. Over a year on hospice, he gradually built up his daily dose of roxanol to 200mg, which he said helped his symptoms of COPD. When I noticed his breathing was unlabored, he was chain-smoking, and rarely used his 0_2, I asked him what the morphine was doing for him. He admitted his COPD symptoms were not the issue, but he had developed an emotional need for the morphine. We were overmedicating him. After much discussion with the team, and naturally some resistance on his part, we scaled him back to extended-release morphine three times a day with a limited, as needed dose of oxycodone for chronic back pain and Ativan. This change was necessary because we could not document his need for the large dose of roxanol and ethically we could not enable his addiction. The MD could not justify the prescriptions.

Over time he did well on this new med regime, but it was very important that we offered him as much ancillary staff as possible. This veteran was a talented painter, so we offered him an art therapist/social worker, a regular social worker, a home health aide daily, a nurse three times a week, a chaplain, and we called the veterans society to schedule visits. Calling upon an extended team, we gave him a great deal of attention and he responded well. His needs were so enormous it was a difficult to understand the void he was trying to fill. His wounds were so deep and his suffering so intense that it was tempting to just give more and more medicine, but what he really responded to was love and attention.

Patients With Young Children

Patients with younger children are another group of patients who may choose less medication because they want to be alert for their children and family and be a parent as long as they can. Offer adjunct, nonnarcotic medication and alternative therapies. They might be open to Reiki, music therapy, added social worker involvement, and very important, early bereavement care for the kids. Choosing to be alert versus totally comfortable may cause them to appear to suffer more. This is not for us to judge. I find parents need to parent, no matter their age, and this need is exacerbated when younger children are involved. Parents know, and need to decide, what is best for their family. I certainly could not know what their children need. The hospice nurse educates and supports despite her discomfort and opinions. The hospice team is critical in these homes.

Patients with Addictions

Others who may have difficulty taking mind-altering meds are those who have had a history of addiction and are frightened of losing control of their sobriety and undoing all the hard work of becoming and remaining clean.

Explain that addiction is physical and psychological and remind them that they probably would not take the med if they were not symptomatic. Add to this that building a tolerance differs from being addicted to a substance. Many patients are hesitant to increase their dose for fear they are becoming addicts. Nursing can assuage these fears by teaching them that eventually most people on a narcotic or sedative for a length of time will develop a tolerance and that this is normal and planned for. It does not mean they are becoming addicted.

"People have a hard time letting go of their suffering. Out of a fear of the unknown, they prefer suffering that is familiar."[39] It seems to me some patients may unconsciously feel the need to suffer, for complex reasons they, or we, cannot understand. I have had experience when patients are in obvious discomfort yet deny themselves adequate comfort meds, or they may resist the effects of the comfort meds and receive no benefit from even very large doses. You may feel powerless seeing a patient suffering, but you may also sense he or she has drawn an impermeable boundary. Notify the team chaplain and social worker for support. Investigate with the patient what may be behind the thinking. Give the family and patients' all options and offer nonnarcotic medication. Offer choices of the lowest doses possible and a range. "We die the way we live" is a slogan you will learn to appreciate. It is very difficult for the hospice RN who feels responsible for his or her patients' discomfort and feels he or she has failed despite her best efforts. Seek support. Very occasionally, no matter what you do, patients will die with stressful symptoms, but it may be the way they need to die.

---

39 Goodreads. Thích Nhất Hạnh. Accessed December 2015. www.goodreads.com.

CHAPTER 9

Preaching

● ● ●

LIKE ARGUING, HOSPICE NURSES CAN be tempted to offer their personal opinions, philosophies, and ideas on faith to patients and families. They may bring these silently to the bedside to help them cope and gain insight, but the beliefs are our own and are not be shared at the bedside. The patients and families have constructed their own belief systems or not. Chogyal Rinpoche said, "We do not push our own 'spiritual formula' to the dying. No one wishes to be rescued with someone else's beliefs. We are not present to convert or push our agenda. We are there to help the person in front of you get in touch with his or her own strength, confidence, faith, and spirituality, that might be."[40] We will not be saving or changing anyone as a hospice nurse, but with our deep sense of caring and our agenda-free approach, we hope to have a positive effect by doing our job with respect for others' choices.

WHEN TO STAND FIRM

Nursing means relinquishing control often, but there are times to stand firm.

For instance, when the patient is failing and absolutely cannot cope at home, either alone or with a caregiver, nurses need to insist on a new plan.

---

40 Rinpoche, *The Tibetan Book of Living and Dying*, 174.

It is a very sad day when someone must leave his or her home. This was probably the hardest thing I did in hospice, because control was stripped completely away from the patient and family. Call the social worker for support to help find a facility, or you can alert the family to discuss possible transfer to a family member's home. Very few people want to leave their homes, especially if it was their one desire was to remain there to die. In these rare situations, the team must take control out of a sincere desire to make the patient more comfortable, safe, and well cared for.

Stand firm when a patient or family member denigrates another team member. Remember the golden rule. Avoid judging a situation you may not fully understand. Defend your colleague by not engaging in the conversation further, and refrain from supporting those doing the denigrating, even if you may not understand or are even surprised by your team member's decisions. Knowing the good quality of your team members, you surmise he or she had a good reason for his or her decision. If the case manager is the one being criticized, it is possible the decision was based on information you do not have. When patients or families show a pattern of being critical of team members, it is known as splitting. It is a form of gathering allies and may temporarily make you feel good, especially if you make a change they like better and they praise your intelligence. Eventually splitting degrades trust among the family and staff because of the inconsistency and derision. There is a good chance at some point you, too, will join the ranks of those maligned, if this is a pattern with this family.

There is a wonderful book by Don Miguel Ruiz called *The Four Agreements* that give us a path for good behavior. The first agreement is "Be Impeccable with Your Word":

> Speak with integrity. Say only what you mean. Avoid using the word to speak against yourself or to gossip about others. Use the power of your word in the direction of truth and love. Impeccable

means "without sin" and a sin is something you do or believe that goes against yourself. It means not speaking against yourself, to yourself or to others. It means not rejecting yourself. To be impeccable means to take responsibility for yourself, to not participate in "the blame game.[41]

Splitting among your colleagues is destructive to the collaboration between the team members. Splitting is a form of gossip that is chiefly derogatory. All of us can be tempted to say, "I can't believe she did that" or "I wouldn't have blah, blah, blah..." When you are tempted to say anything negative about someone, remember Thích Nhất Hạnh's words, "Become like a stick of wood." Your lack of response could be the dose of cold water on the flames of derision. The team needs first to be kind and supportive of one another. Dr. Welch encourages us to have a goal and practice to avoid criticizing other practitioners and their advice, even if we disagree.

---

41 Ruiz. www.goodreads.com (November 2015)

CHAPTER 10

Letting Go—Do We Have To?

● ● ●

I BELIEVE LETTING GO OF our attachments to the people we love and our possessions is one of our greatest tasks in life. Though we are constantly given the opportunity to practice letting go just by watching each moment, breath, and day pass, never to be repeated, we still avoid dealing with the obvious evidence of impermanence. Grieving and letting go can seem so awful that a human will use any device, defense mechanism, or treasure trove of tricks to deny, or at least put off, what is inevitable. In hospice, you will witness many stages of this letting-go process in the patients and families. Patients may understand they have a fatal illness but not acknowledge they are dying, or they may feel determined to beat the disease, hoping for a miracle until their final breath.

Within one family, you will see varying degrees of the process of letting go. Over time, the cloudy lens of denial usually clears, and family members will acknowledge their person is dying. Not always, though. It may take the actual death for them to realize the person was dying. Family members can become angry when a sibling or other family member lags behind in acceptance, or a sibling feels the others are hastening the dying process. You are not in control of their process as it is an individual task. Gradually, people may receive the insights they need just by being present during the patient's decline. Educate and guide them through the dying process. In your own life, you might have had an experience that no one could have told you to get out of, such as a destructive relationship, an unhealthy habit, your baby blanket, or even your old tennies until you were good and ready to do so. We can't rush or cajole people into healing, and letting go is part of healing.

CHAPTER 11

Letting Go of the Outcome and Our Mistakes

● ● ●

PEMA CHÖDRÖN, AN AMERICAN BUDDHIST nun, said, "Let go of all hopes of fruition," meaning let go of the outcome of your work. In genuine self-less service, the server has no needs other than to serve and the outcome released. Sounds lofty, I know. When a nurse releases expectations of how everything will work, the work becomes less torturous.

When you are dedicated to do your best with the team, the outcome is as it should be. This may mean the patient may not reach a peaceful place or appear supremely comfortable. Or he or she may have a lovely death, full of peace and acceptance. It may be that the patient chooses.

The history of the patient's illness and his or her family dynamics provide too many variables for you to predict an ending or for you to hope to be nominated for any awards for a job well done. When we give so much, there may a smidgeon of feeling entitled to some small amount of glory and maybe a little applause. Unless you are a true saint, you can become giddy and puffed up from praise and recognition. Hospice provides such a helpful service, and inevitably you will be stroked and raised to the heavens with a family's expressions of gratitude. It will feel like a good drug—you just can't get enough of that good stuff. Confidence is good, but praise can make a person cocky. When I am in cocky mode, I will make a mistake, forget something, be wrong about a prognosis or a death time, and make other errors. Whenever I have been in this risky and very temporary state, the cosmos goes into emergency mode to bring me right down to ground level, the mud zone. Hospice nursing is humbling. The second you think, "Gosh, I'm good," watch out. As my sister likes to say, "That tether ball is coming around to smack you again in the head."

Besides applause sometimes we (OK, I) just want to be right. I wanted my medicine dose to work perfectly or the patient to die when I said he or she would because I did not want to look bad, and I wanted to maintain his or her family's respect. How's that for evolved thinking and nursing?

Of course, non-saints need affirmation for the work they do. Affirmation can be one form of nourishment, but should not be the sole source. We cannot rely on exhausted and stressed families and patients to buoy our spirits or take care of our emotional needs. We can work on discovering other methods to nurture ourselves besides work. The work will drain us quickly if we need a daily dose of applause, so do the good work and let it go. Become aware of when you feel a need for affirmation and tell yourself it is OK to want some acknowledgement, but you will seek comfort elsewhere. Continue to develop your spiritual life, for this is the most reliable source of comfort. My teacher says, "Put your worries in the lap of the divine." Put your patients and their outcomes there as well.

Letting go of the outcome of each patient's experience can be very difficult for me. When I invest a great deal of time and energy into a family, I *really* want them to have a, it sounds strange, but good experience on hospice. I am not being altruistic, for this hope is not just for them. I squirm saying this, but I know that when things have not gone according to my plan, patient symptoms are unpleasant and not well controlled, or I am wrong about something regarding their care, my ego reacts badly. Yes, I feel badly for the patient, but I also may feel some shame that I might have failed someone. Then it's all about me and my pain. Being egocentric will make this work more painful than it needs to be. If we abandon all hopes of fruition, meaning if we do our best and let the natural course of events flow, we will not feel the distress and responsibility that can plague us as nurses.

Letting go of outcomes also means letting go of our mistakes. I was, and am capable still, of being a real teeth-gnashing nurse. I allowed self-doubt to fester and disable me. I have been at times unhealthy in my anguish over patient and family reactions to me and the outcome of the case. My feeling of responsibility exhausted and disturbed me. Making an error or disappointing a family caused me to feel overwhelming shame. And I did make plenty of mistakes, as my first paragraph indicated. I may even have a reputation for it because when I made a mistake, I fessed up immediately to my administrators. I could not bear steeping in shame and darkness alone, and I felt lonely. I had nurses ask me after one of these disclosures, "Why are you telling us all this?"

When that good, smart hospice nurse friend opted for hospice, we all had to decide who on the team would care for her. After much discussion, my friend decided that I and another nurse on our staff would care for her. I was terrified I would make a mistake, because letting her down during this extremely difficult time would be the ultimate error, the unforgivable. She went on a patient-controlled analgesia pump, and determined as I was not to make a mistake, I *did* miscalculate the drip rate, and she ran out of meds in the wee hours of the morning. I did what I dreaded most of all! She had some narcotic tabs in the home, so she was comfortable. Still, I caused her anxiety, I eroded some trust probably, though she never admitted to it. She was her beautiful, graceful, tactful self and showed no disappointment, but oh how I suffered the shame. I had been so distracted by anxiety that I was not truly concentrating. I had to let this go so that I could continue to care for her with self-respect instead of sopping wet in shame. People who are very ill do not need this type of energy near them. My friend and I talked about it, and she was lovely in her forgiveness. I was lucky she was lovely. Our patients are frequently so unbelievably forgiving and full of grace.

Another hallmark mistake I made was in a home where there were different concentrations of morphine. I made a math error and was giving the wrong concentration to the patient. The patient was fine, though she was getting less morphine than we thought. I was frantically trying to figure out where all the meds went and was wracking my brain, even silently accusing other staff of taking it! I was out on a walk later that day when I realized I did not read the concentration correctly. I made the error. I felt both mortified with guilt and relieved for the mystery's resolution. My first response was an aggressive denial of responsibility with furious attempts to maintain my position of innocence. This frenzy obscured the truth. I had to go to the family to right the wrong I had done, and they were very gracious.

Making mistakes happens, but we should avoid if possible, obsessing about our unworthiness. This takes practice. How seriously you take yourself and how much self-flagellation you enjoy will determine your level of suffering. I read this quote a little too late in my career and life: "You should not burden your mind with anxieties about (your patients). Keep your mind free. Your treatment and service will help them, but not your worrying about them. Worry weakens your power to be useful to them."[42] Do your best. Trust that what needs to happen will.

Knowing patients die the way they live can help nurses let go of the outcome of their work. Even so, I find letting go of results challenging. Early in my hospice career I made the mistake of not sharing the load with my team, so I felt ultraresponsible for my patients' outcomes. When I committed to a patient and his or her family, I assume the responsibility for their well-being and the patient's peaceful death. This had the potential to make me feel either giddily high or saturated with guilt, depending on how well things went. Being at the mercy of others' thought processes, lifestyle choices, and disease processes, I was on constantly shifting ground. Focusing on the outcome wore me down to a nub.

---

42 Welch, *How the Art of Medicine Makes the Science More Effective*, 171.

CHAPTER 12

Seeking Affirmation

● ● ●

IF OUR FEELINGS OF WORTH are lacking, we may try to replenish them by seeking affirmation and attention. This can be an insatiable void to fill. Far from always being altruistic, I have been attention-seeking my whole life. Ask my siblings, and they will concur. They often said, "Peg's just fishing for compliments." I continued this mild form of manipulation to get people to like and acknowledge me. Of course, I often felt others' affirmations were inauthentic because I asked for them. I know I was not being unkind or even unprofessional. It was my level of maturity at the time. I may have been recreating my family scenario where there was a deficit of affirmation, (*sorry, Mom and Dad*). We bring our past into our work.

When we feel whipped by the winds of criticisms, capsized by rejection, or when our feelings of self-worth fluctuate like a small boat on the capricious seas of others' emotions, it might be time to consider finding ways to strengthen and add some substance to our inner ballasts. We can find meaning in many areas of our lives. I believe how we attend to our hunger is a lifelong task. We are working in a healthy manner when we are aware our work is meaningful, we can be at ease when away from it, and we have developed a wholesome life beyond work. According to the ancient healing system of Ayurveda, the word for health is *swastha*, meaning "one who is situated in the self." To me, this is the image of someone who is grounded in the sense of who he or she is, firm in his or her commitments, and has the equanimity and flexibility to allow for the continual flow of life caused by the impermanence of all worldly things.

I find *The Four Agreements* by Don Miguel Ruiz to be an enormously helpful book as long I remember to apply the agreements in a timely manner. One of the four agreements, "Always Do Your Best," is helpful to consider as we learn the art of letting go.

> Your best is going to change from moment to moment; it will be different when you are healthy as opposed to sick. Under any circumstance, simply do your best, and you will avoid self-judgment, self-abuse, and regret. Doing your best means enjoying the action without expecting a reward. The pleasure comes from doing what you like in life and having fun, not from how much you get paid. Enjoy the path traveled and the destination will take care of itself.
>
> Living in the moment and releasing the past helps us to do the best we can in the moment. It allows us to be fully alive right now, enjoying what is present, not worrying about the past or the future.
>
> Have patience with yourself. Take action. Practice forgiveness. If you do your best always, transformation will happen as a matter of course.[43]

Ruiz's second agreement, "Don't Take Anything Personally," also creates space to let go of some of the emotion of the job.

> Nothing others do is because of you. What others say and do is a projection of their own dream. When you are immune to the opinions and actions of others, you won't be the victim of needless suffering. We take things personally when we agree with what others have said. If we didn't agree, the things that others say would

---

43 Ruiz, *The Four Agreements*, page #.

not affect us emotionally. If we did not care about what others think about us, their words or behavior could not affect us. Even if someone yells at you, gossips about you, harms you or yours, it still is not about you! Their actions and words are based on what they believe in their personal dream.[44]

Families and patients are too overloaded, stressed, and ultrafocused with their tasks at hand to protect your tender psyche. Families may respond blandly to you because they have no energy to do otherwise. Perhaps you remind them of someone, maybe they don't like blondes, or your sense of humor (I *told* you to cool it), or your style of nursing. They may not appreciate all your questions or new people being in their home. I wasn't a good fit in some homes. Being overly sensitive to people's opinions or reactions to you will only wear you out, so that is why I love the second agreement. I just have a problem remembering it.

Ruiz's third agreement, "Don't Make Assumptions," also helps us in our work and day-to-day life.

Find the courage to ask questions and to express what you really want. Communicate with others as clearly as you can to avoid misunderstandings, sadness, and drama. With just this one agreement, you can completely transform your life. When we make assumptions, it is because we believe we know what others are thinking and feeling. We believe we know their point of view, their dream. We forget that our beliefs are just our point of view based on our belief system and personal experiences and have nothing to do with what others think and feel. Take action, and be clear to others about what you want or do not want; do not gossip and make assumptions about things others tell you. Respect other points of view and avoid arguing just to be right. Respect yourself and be

---

44 Ruiz, *The Four Agreements*, page #.

honest with yourself. Stop expecting the people around you to know what is in your head.[45]

I have had difficulty developing that thick skin of protection, and I have a reputation for being overly sensitive. I wish I could take the advice one father gave his daughter, "Be like a duck and let the water just roll off your feathers." I stink at that. Because I am more like a sponge than a duck, I have times when I need to dialogue with my team for a better perspective. With luck, they will remind me of what I did correctly and unravel the facts to help me face where I may have screwed up. Instead of convincing others of your innocence and gathering allies, be very honest with yourself. You are going to make errors, you just are. Learn how to forgive yourself and pick yourself up.

Dr. Welch reminds us that a patient or family emotional crisis should not become our crisis:

> "Empathy is good, but over-identification with the patients' feelings may cause us to lose our perspective. Losing our perspective, we lose our connection with ourselves, our source, patients and family."[46]
>
> Your aim can be to be the calm person who is able to keep perspective and help others remain grounded.

---

45 Ruiz, *The Four Agreements*, page #.
46 Welch, *How the Art of Medicine Makes the Science More Effective*, 172.

CHAPTER 13

We Die the Way We Live

● ● ●

THERE ARE THE FIGHTERS, THE loners, the driven, the introverts, extroverts, the calm ones, the worriers, the fearful, the anxiety-ridden, and everyone in between. No one changes just because they are dying. I think personality traits are exaggerated in the process of dying. Worriers are not going to relax just because you tell them to. Are you able to stop worrying when someone tells you to? Become familiar with your patients' character traits. You can ask the family, "What's Jane like as a person?" Often family are happy to tell you what the patient will not. The patient might tell you a few of the quirks they like about themselves. Consider giving more emotional support to those who are known to be highly anxious. Assist with details of care for those who are detail oriented. Offer low-dose antianxiety medicine for those with anxiety. Give space for the fighters to fight. Assist the meticulous with the funeral plans they feel compulsive about completing. Try not to push medicine on a stoic. Go with their flows. This can be summed up with "meet the patient where they are."

We want to understand our patients beyond superficialities, and the obvious and enjoyable way to do this is by spending relaxed time listening to them. We are lucky in hospice care that this is a vital part of the job. If death appears imminent, we might need to ask family sooner than later: "Does Joe typically admit to pain? How does Emily express her needs? Does Marion like to be touched? Does John tend to like some commotion or quiet?" Even if you have been with the patient for some time, try not to assume you know your patient so well that you feel you know just what he or she needs. I know I loathe it when people tell me what they think I need, even those close to me. Out of all the people in the patient's room, you probably know the patient the least.

Some patients will fight to live while some can't wait to die. "Why doesn't God want me? I want to die!" a ninety-five-year-old said to me. She had a great sense of humor; she said she had a very good relationship with God and was ready to go. Another said to me, "I don't want to go because I want to know what they are going to say at my funeral, and I want it to go well." Some have FOMO, or fear of missing out, and simply do not want to leave the lovefest that often occurs at the hospice bedside. Some want to stay as much in control as possible. One spouse told me her husband obsessively focused on his funeral, despite his extremely poor condition, and would not die until the plans were perfect. He planned the last scene of his service where everyone would gather outside and watch helium balloons that had a small amount of his ashes be set free over the treetops while his favorite song played. He had always been a planner, so creating and having his family commit to his plan helped him die peacefully.

My mother-in-law was as tough as boiled owl according to her son Roger. At nearly ninety-four and maybe sixty-five pounds, she kept trying to feed herself ("I need protein," she said) and give herself fluids ("I don't want to get dehydrated") even though she was weak as a baby bird. Her will to live and a lifetime resolve to fight through all obstacles kept her alive far beyond anyone's predictions. She astonished her family and the staff at the nursing home.

CHAPTER 14

A Bit More on Rejection

● ● ●

FITTING IN, OR NOT

PATIENT AND FAMILY EMOTIONS RUN the gamut under the stress of grave illness, anger being the more difficult to manage because of what it may trigger in us. Occasionally, we seem to have a bull's-eye on our foreheads, and we may become a temporary target for some of this anger. Some nurses may feel rejected or submerge themselves in guilt and self-doubt based on their own family history and level of self-esteem. The lower the self-esteem, the more painful it is. It is especially difficult when the family or patient ask the nurse not to return. Refer to the beginning of this book. Looking back at the situation, I realized the family was angry long before I arrived. They were angry at the disease and loss, but it sure felt personal at the time. "When a person's speech is full of anger, it is because he or she suffers deeply."[47]

Sometimes we just aren't a good fit with a family. We might even get the boot from a family. It is important to scrutinize your activity because their observations may be legitimate. I had to ask myself if I was sensitive enough to the family who asked me not to return, if I had missed the obvious, or failed them in some way. I know I was trying very hard, maybe too hard. After you have put yourself through a trial by judge and jury,

---

47 Thích Nhất Hạnh

it is helpful to remember Ruiz's suggestions: take nothing personally and never assume anything, such as you are worthless and should immediately leave your nursing career. Eventually, I had to let the whole rejection scene go because there was nothing else I could do. The end product was never going to change. Now when I think of those times, I do not suffer, and I can share the story honestly. I love the Irish saying "When the horse is dead, get off." (Thank you, Sheila C.)

There is a movie titled *Everyone Loves a Good Train Wreck* so who doesn't want to hear another story about my getting fired by a family? A good friend's sister came on hospice, and we all thought it would be great if I could care for her. I knew the patient only a bit more than an acquaintance. Things were going along fine, or so I thought, when one day they told me they were going to have another RN provide care per the patient's choice. Oh, that hurt. I was given some rationale, but what I believe it came down to was my trying to get this girl to talk...about her feelings, about dying. And she was too uncomfortable going there. Now I understand that just because I think we should discuss this heavy stuff doesn't mean anyone else does. Maybe when I am dying, I will not want to discuss it either. My friend's sister may have wanted to think about living. If so, I don't blame her for getting me out of there. I reeled for a while after this, and it did affect my relationship with her sister for a bit, but I eventually got off that horse too.

CHAPTER 15

Being There

● ● ●

To PARAPHRASE JEAN WATSON, NURSES are encouraged to practice loving-kindness and equanimity with what she calls "caring consciousness." They instill faith and hope by being authentically present with their patients. By cultivating their own spiritual practices and learning the significance of going beyond ego, they can develop and sustain a helping-trusting, authentic caring relationship. Nurses support their patients' expression of positive and negative feelings.

> Nurses create a healing environment on all levels, physical as well as non-physical, a subtle environment of energy and consciousness, whereby wholeness, beauty and comfort, dignity and peace are potentiated.[48]

After nursing tasks are completed and the patient's symptoms are well managed, sitting quietly with the patient and family is wonderful medicine. It takes practice to feel comfortable with someone who is dying. In hospice, I like to use an old CPR practice. When a potential rescuer initially happens upon someone who has collapsed, they are first to look, listen, and feel. At the bedside we can relax our clinical perspective and look with a soft gaze at the person in the bed. Deeply perceive them. Listen to

---

48 Jean Watson, PhD, RN HNC, FAAN, " Intentionality and Caring-Healing Consciousness: A Practice of Transpersonal Nursing." *Holistic Nurse Practice* 16, no. 4 (2002): 13.

their stories and feel the breadth and depth of them. Listen to the silence. Feel their stories and their current situations as well as who they were.

Sometimes simply sitting at the bedside can be emotionally uncomfortable. I love this teaching of Thích Nhất Hạnh:

> When you feel overwhelmed, you're trying too hard. That kind of energy does not help the other person and it does not help you. You should not be too eager to help right away. There are two things: to be and to do. Don't think too much about to do—to be is first. To be peace. To be joy. To be happiness. And then to do joy, to do happiness—on the basis of being. So, first you have to focus on the practice of being. Being fresh. Being peaceful. Being attentive. Being generous. Being compassionate. This is the basic practice. It's like if the other person is sitting at the foot of a tree. The tree does not do anything, but the tree is fresh and alive. When you are like that tree, sending out waves of freshness, you help to calm down the suffering in the other person.[49]

I love this quote by Cicely Saunders, the great pioneer of the hospice movement in Britain: "I once asked a man who knew he was dying what he needed above all in those who were caring for him. He said, 'For someone to look as if they are trying to understand me.'"[50] Care enough to try.

"Human Life is a Sacred thing," said Swami Paramananda. Since death is part of life, then death must be sacred as well. To me, death must be spiritual for all beings, not just the "believers."

> "Peaceful death is really an essential human right, more essential perhaps even than the right to vote or the right to justice; it is a

---

49 Thich Naht Hanh
50 Rinpoche, *The Tibetan Book of Living and Dying*, 176.

right on which all religious traditions tell us, a great deal depends for the well-being and spiritual future of the dying person."[51]

There will be difficult patients who challenge our compassion, and we might feel we cannot love them or even like them. You will care for those whose histories repulse you. Sogyal Rinpoche offers two methods in which you can release the love within you toward the dying person:

> First, look at the dying person in front of you and think of that person as just like you, with the same needs, the same fundamental desire to be happy and avoid suffering, the same loneliness, the same fear of the unknown, the same secret areas of sadness, the same half-acknowledged feelings of helplessness.
>
> The second way, and I have found this even more powerful, is to put yourself directly and unflinchingly in the dying person's place. Imagine that you are on that bed before you, facing your death. Imagine that you are there in pain and alone. Then really ask yourself: What would you most need? What would you most like? What would you really wish from this friend in front of you?[52]

Further along this chapter, he said:

> So, compassion reveals itself yet again as your greatest resource and your greatest protection. They are actively helping you to develop your compassion, and so purify and heal yourself. For me, every dying person is a teacher, giving all those who help them a chance to transform themselves through developing their compassion.[53]

A beautiful, physical practice most patients love that feels sacred to me is the simple act of foot soaking, and if not soaking, then gently washing. It

---

51 Rinpoche, *The Tibetan Book of Living and Dying*, 186.
52 Ibid.,175.
53 Rinpoche, *The Tibetan Book of Living and Dying*, 178

brings us to our knees if the patient is seated and offers us an opportunity to simply serve them. Plus, feet are an oft-neglected part of the body, rarely visited as other parts seem to get all the attention. It is relaxing for both you and the patient, allows opportunity to talk quietly as the feet soak and the patient feels respected and cared for. Clean, warm feet feel sublime. And clean socks. Not to make a comparison, but I think Jesus liked to wash others' feet and put clean sandals on them.

A nurse brings his or her personality, gifts, and delightful idiosyncrasies to the bedside of his or her patients. Some days we may be bursting with vigor and enthusiasm for life, full of (coffee?) beans. When entering a home though, we must bottle some of our vitality, at least temporarily. Maybe you can uncork it later. It is important to enter a home calmly to be able to perceive the vibes of the home. Use your internal Geiger counter. The environment might be subdued and calm, tense, chaotic or loud, or may change depending on the personalities present. You may find you need to be the calming presence.

Patients and families have different tastes in nurses. Some may not appreciate a laid-back nurse, preferring one with lots of pizzazz. Some people appreciate questions regarding their emotional well-being and some prefer a straightforward, clinical approach. We may feel at home with some families and awkward in others. Connection can vary. Occasionally, you will need to surrender your patient to the sort of nurse he or she prefers, which happened to me. It might hurt a little, but in the long run, everyone will benefit.

You will need to evaluate the tone each time you enter any home, even if you know the family well. As you build a trusting relationship with your patients and families, you might be able to be your bawdy, uproarious self, but you need your sensitivity gauge working consistently. The rowdy home might be subdued the next day, and you will need to morph yourself into that quiet person. I recall these words of Friedrich Nietzsche, "Learn to see...accustom the eye to calmness, to patience, and to allow things to come up to it."

There are times when you have given every medicine, discussed obvious issues, tried all positions, and still the patient seems distressed. Often this is spiritually based distress. It can be as challenging as physical pain and must treated as promptly. Though the hospice chaplain focuses on spiritual issues, nurses often need to assist people emotionally or spiritually on the spot. Besides manifesting physically, spiritual issues may arise during a conversation. You might notice topics blending like watercolor on canvas. A clinical discussion of comfort measures can merge into care concerns about sibling rivalry, God, forgiveness, love, and letting go. This is beautiful, often challenging landscape to venture into with them. It is helpful to have a canvas large and open enough to support the fluctuation of emotions as people go through this experience. If you feel overwhelmed, encourage them to speak with the chaplain as soon as possible.

According to Atul Gawande:

> As people become aware of the finitude of their life, they do not ask for much. They do not seek more riches. They do not seek more power. They ask only to be permitted, insofar as possible, to keep shaping the story of their life in the world—to make choices and sustain connections to others according to their own priorities.[54]

As part of the hospice team, nurses need to be open to and encourage patient sharing. It could be their first or last time they tell it, or the thousandth. Always respect the story.

I believe that sitting at a bedside, deeply perceiving and listening, is powerful medicine for everyone present, including the nurse. When you feel

---

54 Gawande, *Being Mortal*, 146.

perplexed about how to handle a patient's spiritual questions, you may find sitting quietly provides the time needed for him or her to relax enough to talk. Give your patient complete attention. From this place, you both may be surprised by the depth of wisdom that emerges and some old, and new, truths are realized. "The sources of healing and awareness are deep within each of us, and your task is never under any circumstances to impose your beliefs, but to enable them to find these within themselves."[55] The art of sitting quietly together is simple yet profound.

Dr. Claudia Welch gives us a way to be with people who are deep in a struggle or grieving. "Stand under the waterfall with them." Simply be present. Say nothing. Words will often fail us or fail others. Words of support for one person may aggravate another; therefore, our best support is being quiet sometimes. There can be profound communication by just standing with someone. The greatest needs during the dying process seem to be for comfort and companionship, so we need to build our capacity to just sit quietly with them.

Dr. Welch said:

> If we can communicate on a deeper level than words, the exact words may not matter as much. When we don't let suffering divide us, and we commit to hearing, seeing, and feeling more deeply, we can meet there, in that place that words can't reach-that horrible, real, sometimes grace-filled, beautiful, tender and exquisite reality.[56]

If the patient is unable or unwilling to participate in any way, your own spiritual practice, your faith in something larger is a strong support for you at the bedside. When at a loss for something to say, or do, silently pray, meditate, or invoke the figure or energy whose sacred power you

---

55 Rinpoche, *The Tibetan Book of Living and Dying*, 211.
56 Welch, *Being Mortal*, 127.

believe in. You could call on the enlightened beings with whom you have a connection. Using all your devotion and faith, Rinpoche says, "See them in glory above the patient, gazing down at them with love, and pouring down light and blessing on them, purifying them and all their past karma and present agony."[57] These are the heights we could reach with our intentions and compassion and another reason to cultivate a relationship with a greater being or power—not only for ourselves, but with the purpose of helping others through our intentions and compassion.

The peaceful practice of Reiki, or any other energy healing methods, are helpful tools for being present at the bedside of the dying. When all physical means of nursing have been done, these skills can be soothing and relaxing. Maybe we could use it more often than waiting for when all else fails. Sitting silently by a bed with hands either placed lightly on or hovering over a patient may appear a little weird to some folks, so a simple explanation is best. "Reiki is a 'hands-off' or light 'hands-on' method of offering 'good-vibes' to people, of conducting healing energy to the patient through yourself."[58] You will be surprised at how willing people are to receive this sort of treatment. I've had patients and family members go to sleep quickly during Reiki. One woman said, "Don't ever stop doing that." Some eagerly await their next Reiki session. Some maintain they feel nothing but want you to continue, and others say, "That's enough." You will know what to do.

I encourage you to investigate Reiki or Healing Touch or another form of hands-on healing. These are good to have in your toolkit of ways to add to people's experience. Plus, you can do this sort of healing on yourself.

I recently read a book by a young girl who was very ill with cancer. She was about fourteen years old when she wrote this. She had already spent

---

57 Rinpoche, *The Tibetan Book of Living and Dying*, 211.
58 The International House of Reiki, Frans Steine, accessed in 2016, www.ihreiki.com.

an enormous amount of time in hospitals for her treatments. This is what she feels makes a good nurse, and I could not resist including this here.

> They can get blood out of your veins on the first try.
> They don't wake you up in the morning.
> They know how to put on and take off duoderm without taking your skin off.
> They don't talk to me as if I'm a baby.
> They don't wake me up when I am sleeping.
> They are patient even when I am grumpy
> They listen to my requests with respect.
> They don't wake me up![59]

COMPASSION

I remember the Dalai Lama saying to a huge audience in Boston, "If you want others to be happy, practice compassion. If you want to be happy, practice compassion."

In *The Tibetan Book of Living and Dying*, Sogyal Rinpoche states, "The first quality you need to manifest when present at the bedside of someone who is dying, and with their family, is that of compassion." Compassion implies respect. Embedded in respect is your intention for the highest good for all. "At every moment in our lives we need compassion, but what more urgent moment could there be than when we are dying?"[60]

Nurses as well as doctors can practice the art of medicine. Dr. Welch discusses several qualities central to the art of medicine—humility, confidence, healthy communication skills, and empathy—but she feels compassion rises to the top:

---

59 Ester Earl, 81.
60 Rinpoche, *The Tibetan Book of Living and Dying*, 206.

Compassion seems to be both a seed and a fruit. It seems to be a seed that, when nourished, yields deeper knowledge, richer experience, more dexterous medical intuition, and a purer heart. At the same time, it also seems a natural fruit of cultivating these four qualities. If we can do nothing else—if we can't arrive at an elegant diagnosis, if we are at a loss for an effective treatment plan, if we are confused about our prescriptions, at least our patients will benefit from compassion. And when we feel it for them, we are experiencing it ourselves.[61]

But what is compassion? According to Dr. Welch, compassion "may not be something we feel for others. It may just be something we feel. It may be more of a space or room we choose to enter, where we focus on the Good, the Real, the Stable, the True inside ourselves, moment to moment, and attempt to perceive it in others."[62]

Darn it all. This means we must really understand compassion for ourselves and develop loving self-care habits. *Don't you hate that?* And we must work on this daily, over and over. One day we get it, one day we don't. Some days we need to cut ourselves some slack, other days we need to tighten the reins. Life is confusing.

JUDGMENT

"What is love? Love is the absence of judgment."—Dalai Lama

It is easy to judge our patients simply by their address or phone exchange within a town. As we approach the house, we evaluate its condition. We walk in and might experience an unpleasant smell, a thick cigarette fog, or walk into a dark, cavernous, hazardous falling-hoarded-objects zone.

---

61 Welch, *Being Mortal*, 234.
62 Ibid., 234.

Homes may not reach our standards for cleanliness even if our standards are low. It is going to happen, and you might want to drive away. You can't leave, but you can opt to at least work on and even erase judgment. We can redirect our focus to the care of the patient and family, realizing they are suffering human beings in need of great support. It is possible they have had a hard life or have no emotional or physical means to improve their situation. Judging thoughts arise beyond our control. Note your judgment, but give it no weight, no attention. "We feed what we focus on" is a favorite saying of Dr. Welch. Imagine these thoughts as cars on a train and let the train pass on by, or imagine the thoughts as dandelion fluff in the breeze. Let them go. Replace the thought with one of compassion, soft and kind. Remember, you too will most likely need this sort of intimate care. Remind yourself that this is their home, and they love being there. It is also good to realize opinions on cleanliness are subjective, and someday, or currently, someone might think *you* are a messy hoarder.

According to Dr. Welch, judgment is the opposite of compassion. "When our senses are obstructed by ill will and judgment, we cloud our ability to perceive reality as it truly is."[63] Judging others alienates us from them and even from ourselves. Being critical of others may justify ourselves, but at the same time we turn our backs and hearts on goodness and mercy, the two qualities we all crave. As with impatience, when we judge we throw away opportunities to love. A physician who cowrote original medical textbooks thousands of years ago said, "You should not think ill of patients even at the cost of your own life."[64] A tall order, but nevertheless one to strive for.

Thousands of years ago, humans needed to judge their immediate environment to survive. They lived in fight or flight mode with hungry, enormously toothed animals lurking about and the daily stress of hunting for food and living in the elements. Our environments do not have the same

---

63 Welch, *Being Mortal*, 235.
64 Ibid., 235.

hazards as our ancestors. Now we are more frightened of feeling rejected by not having texts responded to, concerned with how many likes to our brilliant comments we get on Facebook, how the stock market is doing with our meager retirement fund, and how many chemical toxins assault us daily. There is always the realistic fear of driving at high speeds while everyone else is distracted on their phones, or swatting the kids in the backseat who are fighting and watching a violent DVD. Our ability to judge continues to support our navigation in our environment, but it may also hinder our ability to connect to it in a calm and loving way.

I admit I am a harsh judge of myself and others. It may even come more easily than a loving thought, ugly as that sounds. However, constantly judging others makes me feel tense, dark, and unkind. This in turn causes me to feel saturated and depleted. I imagine judgment even appears dark, sticky, and stuck in my body, like an illness. Even Dr. Welch, whom I consider close to enlightened, said, "I have failed at this (judging) more times than I can count. The impulse to judge others, in a myriad of small ways, is insidious, and the fight against it can be long, but in my experience, it is one worth fighting for."[65] Strive to be aware of this energy when you are with your patients. I feel a sense of freedom when I lighten up on people and even on myself. It is much easier to soften and expand the thinking than to rationalize, measure, and criticize. I also wonder how well I am collaborating with folks if I limit them with my judgment. I squelch the flow of working with others by being unloving. Judging makes everything smaller, darker, and keeps us stuck.

---

65 Welch, *Being Mortal*, 235.

CHAPTER 16

Compliance

● ● ●

HEARING THE WORDS *COMPLIANCE* AND *appropriate* causes my hackles to rise, especially when describing me or hospice patients. I feel it is patronizing to set a standard for someone we hardly know who is in a dire situation. Furthermore, we must believe we are superior to set the standard. It is easy to label a patient noncompliant when we are annoyed with him or her for not doing what we ask. Our egos are hurt. Ask yourself how well you comply with rules and advice and then wonder how it would feel if someone wrote in your chart that you were noncompliant or inappropriate. Have you always finished your four times a day, ten-day course of antibiotics? In hospice care we do not need to use these two words because no one needs to comply with anything. The only rule to follow is that we must respect the patient and family and create an atmosphere of peace. One can wonder what appropriate behavior is when we are dying. I do not feel there can be a script for this. When a patient is noncompliant with their medicine regime, engage them in a discussion about it. The meds might make them feel crummy, or they might loathe or cannot swallow medicine. Discuss possible interactions or repercussions, and let the doctor know the patient's decision. Be flexible with what alternatives might exist. Come up with twenty ideas. It's all OK. People do not misbehave in hospice. They are not children. People are going to make what you consider to be poor decisions. We are not the big boss. I read somewhere recently, "They are not giving you a hard time. They are having a hard time." I believe it was written regarding patients with dementia, but it still applies.

Believe it or not, a caregiver might have a better idea than you due to his or her familiarity with the patient. There is no right or wrong way to do things provided no one gets hurt or neglected. Avoid getting into a urinating contest with people. If your suggestions were ignored, respect their ideas and decisions. If you push too hard, you may end up eating more of that tough black bird.

There are rare cases of sexual inappropriateness, and we need to set boundaries and rely on the team. Regarding drug diversion, we need to be firm, but most cases of labeling are possibly instances of labeling of our own. The patient deserves better.

I struggle over the words *patient* and *impatient*. We strive to be loving, kind, and patient with our patients and families, but when we are impatient, we can know we have work to do on ourselves. Feeling impatience signals that we may be feeling superior, have an agenda either for ourselves or the situation, and that we have lost touch with the person in front of us. Impatience has an authoritarian ring to it. Impatience is our experience, but it has nothing to do with the patient. Another person in the same situation may not feel impatient. It is up to us to let go of these judging thoughts. The use of phrases such as "making space for" and "allowing time for them to discover answers for themselves" may alleviate impatience. We are not teachers with all the answers, but guides with open agendas. Swami Paramananda said, "When we are impatient we throw away our opportunities."

CHAPTER 17

Personal Disclosures

● ● ●

IT BENEFITS THE NURSE TO be selective in the amount of personal information to share with patients and families. I would consider sharing only brief, helpful comments and stories about your own life. We wish to add to patient and family experience. We do not need to talk about our issues at home, like the dissolution of a relationship, our children's illnesses, our overloaded schedules, our fatigue, or our own illnesses. When you describe your stresses, you subtly ask for support, affirmation, even alliances, from very vulnerable and weary people. Take those sorts of complaints to your good friends or family if they can stand it.

CHAPTER 18

Love?

● ● ●

WE OCCASIONALLY EXPERIENCE FEELING LOVE in our role as a hospice nurse because we often meet extraordinarily devoted families and patients. They will astound and amaze us. In most humble of homes, I see the best of humanity. I can erase a week's worth of horrible world news in a minute in just one of my patients' homes.

We are drawn into the intimacy of the family. We are often saluted, valued, and adored. People call us angels. They say they can't make it without us. They believe and tell us they need us. Sometimes they say they even worship us. We know we are not angels by a long shot. We are doing work we love. Though the families are not intending to, all the stroking and adoration can easily seduce us. We feel so darn worthwhile, so needed, even loved. We can feel we love them too, especially if we can be very much at ease with them, or perhaps if this warm and fuzzy, beautiful family stuff was lacking in our own upbringing.

This is all wonderful, but you probably know where I am going with this. Everyone is feeling the love, but, my dear nurse, it is temporary. You are practicing compassion for another human and this feels very loving. This is probably not a long-lasting friendship. I have tried to maintain some friendships with a spouse or a patient's children, because I truly enjoyed them. It didn't last, partly because our focal point, the patient, really was the glue for the relationship. You might find there is not so much to talk about after a while. Consider your other friendships and the balance, the give and take, needed to maintain a friendship. This may not be true of the friendship with the family. It may be more one-sided. This does not diminish the goodness or love you felt during your time with them. Though short-lived, it is still a remarkable, valuable experience for all involved.

The other issue is that we are not to maintain friendships with our clients while employed with the hospice.

A family member may want to continue the relationship with you because you are a connection to the person who died. It is hard for families to say yet another goodbye. You have all shared some very intimate experiences and this creates a feeling of closeness. Saying goodbye to families is difficult, but soon enough you will have another admission to distract you.

Going to the wake or funeral is very helpful to gain closure, and the families deeply appreciate you showing up. It is a way to stand under the waterfall with them. I never said anything intelligent or even intelligible at a wake, so I decided the best thing to do is smile and give them a hug. But do go if you can.

And sometimes you feel nothing. This can surprise you. I was concerned I had a personality disorder because sometimes amid human suffering I felt nothing. I felt separate. You can expect to feel nothing at times, but it does not mean you are crazy or subhuman. It is merely self-protection, a withdrawal from overload of emotion. I think each of us has a limit, or we limit ourselves to how much we are capable of managing. It is because we feel that we go to non-feeling. It's like choosing to go into denial. We catch a glimpse of the pain and decide to back away. I think it is normal and temporary. You will be equally surprised how one day someone touches your hand and you break into tears. Don't worry, the emotions are still there. We just might need to tuck them away at times. The hospice nurses I have run this by have all occasionally experienced this lack of feeling.

I find that an antidote to feeling nothing is to expose myself daily to beauty. I put myself in natural settings like the woods, the garden, the water, or gazing at snowfall. Sometimes I listen to soothing music. The simplest chord, or a leaf backlit just so, can release feelings gently and help me regain access to my emotions. Perhaps exposing myself to music or the natural world simply lets me reconnect with myself.

CHAPTER 19

The Changing Nature of the Work

• • •

THE NEED FOR FLEXIBILITY AS a hospice nurse cannot be overemphasized. You benefit from understanding that nothing on earth is permanent. A patient's status can change in a moment, and you will need to shift gears, drive fifty miles to his or her home, and stay with the patient three hours longer than anticipated. Patients die when you do not expect it. Another nurse's patient will die, and you need to do the pronouncement in a home you have never been to.

Always use pencil to do your daily schedule. If the office scheduler observes you writing down your lovely four-patient day in pen, he or she will smile and then dismantle your schedule pronto. You might think schedulers are cruel and out to get you personally, but fate does it to all hospice nurses. To avoid frustration, say to thyself that this schedule I see before me is just a loose guideline guaranteed to be messed with.

One of the most important things I tell patients and families is, "Wake up each day without expectations for how your loved one will be, or how you will feel." When the family or patient is hoping for improvement or expecting decline and the expected does not happen, it wears them down quickly.

Educate patients and families about reality of the roller-coaster ride of illness. Symptoms can be deceiving and can change day to day, sometimes minute to minute. There is a phrase aptly called saw-tooth decline. This is a helpful visual and describes how people generally go through their dying process. During a long course, a patient might improve, then decline a bit, and then plateau for a few months. Short term, the patient can feel well in the morning and struggle more in the afternoon or evening. They can have a rapid downhill turn and then plateau over the next few days, or vice versa. There is no set pattern to dying. Like delivering a baby, the outcome is the same, but the delivery process has its own story.

I have a friend who recently went through the difficult saw-tooth process. Her husband had end-stage dementia and developed a urinary tract infection. Since she was the health care proxy, she called me asking if she should take the option of antibiotics. Following a discussion of pros and cons, she decided not to treat the UTI. She expected him to die within the week according to his symptoms and began to prepare for this. She had been processing this grief and steeling herself for his death for the fourteen years since her husband was diagnosed. During this decision-making he seemed to be entering the next and last phase of his dying process. He was bedbound, agitated, and not eating. However, the next morning her husband was alert and hungry. He was no longer agitated, ate well, and was even ambulatory. My friend was expecting a decline and naturally immersed herself in prepping for his imminent death. Her husband lasted a month longer, and it was difficult for my friend to dial her energy back toward chronic caregiving mode. She had been saying goodbye for too long and was weary.

My own father tried to teach me this lesson as well. At one point near the end of his life, his respiratory rate was six per minute and he was minimally responsive. We siblings had gathered from all over the country to say goodbye. One morning while we were sitting in the living room, Dad, the most modest person of all time, shuffled out of his room naked using a chair as a walker. I remember my unloving, angry response to this. I had already said goodbye. Many times. It was very difficult to shift gears back to the exhausting work of caring for a very ill man. I wanted him to die now. I had to get back to my life. I was supposed to work Christmas day, and how do you get someone to replace you on Christmas? Then my siblings got mad at me for wanting Dad to die and for being mad at him when he was so ill. The whiplash of emotion during these patient rallies can be exhausting and frustrating for everyone. I don't think Dad was feeling the whiplash—he seemed quite content to be naked in the kitchen as he searched for a little piece of bacon and a pickle to snack on. If I had not had expectations for his course for dying, I may not have been set on his dying on my time and my agenda. It's that agenda thing getting in the way again.

Then there is my own mother-in-law. Ninety-four years old, seemingly near death. Hotshot hospice nurse that I am, I called for the gathering of the masses (of family) for the goodbyes, and you know how this went. I was wrong again. She rallied from her near death and began eating large amounts of food. Sometimes you just can't know how it is going to go, even when it appears clear to you.

We may try, but we often cannot predict a patient's course. Even when a patient appears very nearly dead, gray, cold, even mottled, he or she may continue to live days or weeks beyond our predictions. People can live on just small amounts of air for an astonishing amount of time. They can appear so thin as to be translucent. Too many times I have prepared a family for a death, and they gather from far away. Before I know it, the patient is eating French toast and bacon and I am eating crow...again. For some reason, I think that in my great wisdom I can still predict a death. Time and again I am proven wrong, so may I suggest that you try to resist the temptation. (Of course, there were plenty of times I was right.)

Patients can also have a sudden event that will radically change their course. Falls can change the game in seconds. People tend to have more than one disease, and an unexpected exacerbation can erupt. I have had relatively stable hospice patients who seemed to be in a slow decline (though we avoid those two words in hospice) and the team was wondering how we could recertify them. They end up having a surprising, unpredictable ending, sometimes if they are lucky, near their recertification date. A patient with end-stage lung disease developed a gastrointestinal bleed and died within days. A cardiac patient fell and broke her hip and then seemed to will her death by the next morning. A patient with dementia developed a pneumonia, or a UTI. One thirty-year-old cancer patient had a cardiac arrest. Teaching the family about the unpredictable nature of the dying process and the likelihood for surprises helps them cope.

CHAPTER 20

Drug Diversion

● ● ●

DRUG DIVERSION IS RARE, BUT can happen both in homes where you least expect it in and in those that will not surprise you. In some cases, I was willing to give the patient and family the benefit of the doubt until I realized the drugs were disappearing much faster than they should be. You will need all the help you can get from your team in these cases because of our responsibility to keep the patient, family, and drug supply safe and the complex nature of addiction.

After you are sure it is not in fact your error, you can voice your concern. You could say, "Wow, yesterday there were thirty cc's in this bottle and today there are two cc's. Joe said he is uncomfortable and claims he only had two doses. Can you help me understand this?" It is pointless to accuse anyone because it could create a volatile scene that the patient does not need to be part of (assuming the patient is not the party in question). Plus, you will not be able to prove anything. Provide the home with a lockbox with a decent lock. I had one patient, an active drug addict, who laughed at my little lock, saying, "A kindergartener could get into that." Tell the family we often provide a lockbox when there are narcotics in the home to keep the meds organized and accounted for. Usually there is someone to trust in the home. When there is only one person to trust in the home, I have had to tape keys to the lockboxes under couches or hide them in other creative places. One option is to hang them on lanyards around a family member's neck so only that family member can have access to the box. You can also have meds available just for one week and have prefilled, labeled syringes. Mark the bottles with dates and amounts, and create a user-friendly medication log. Let people know you are keeping close tabs on all medicine. Increase the frequency of nursing visits for a while. If the losses are egregious, you can tell the family you will be involving the police. It doesn't feel good to say this, but it's a powerful and effective intervention.

If the patient has been misusing his or her medicine, we need to investigate physical and emotional issues—but we do not withhold comfort measures. We work with the doctor and continue to administer appropriate doses of medication. We must be careful not to push the patient into withdrawal. We cannot deprive anyone of comfort medicine because of a history of abuse or even current use of a substance. An active drug user or alcoholic experiences pain like anyone else. Their emotional distress related to their terminal illness may be even more severe than the nonaddict because of lack of resolution over a tough past and an inability to deal with emotional life. They may have isolated themselves or been estranged from family and friends resulting in a depleted support system. All patients must be respected, even with their addictions. Try to withhold judgment. If we peek at ourselves, I will wager few of us can say we do not have an addiction to something. How aggressively did you seek your coffee this morning? There is a wonderful North American Indian saying, "Do not judge another until you understand their family seven years back and seven years forward." We cannot begin to understand what another has gone through. We all have our battles, scars, and crosses to bear. We cannot change people's habits, but we should be careful not to enable them.

CHAPTER 21

Dementia

● ● ●

"There is no way into presence except through a Love exchange."

—RUMI

ROUGHLY 20 PERCENT OF HOSPICE patients fall under the category of dementia though they have a different hospice diagnosis now. Per the new regulations, we now use diagnoses such as "protein malnutrition," since this is typically what a patient with dementia (PWD) will die of. Caring for these patients can be stressful for other reasons than symptom control and behavior issues. Sometimes there seems to be nothing to do for them other than maintenance care or sitting silently at the bedside. I know I have felt at a loss for a task to do at the bedside of someone who is vaguely present or nonresponsive and feel like I am just logging time with him or her. We take vital signs, auscultate lungs, check their skin, and give a report to the RN on duty. We need to chart carefully on patients with dementia, and sometimes we are repetitive in our entries, which we dislike, and so does Medicare. Logging time is not such a bad thing if you focus on the patient instead of looking at your Facebook page on your phone or checking personal e-mail. Sitting quietly at the bedside is where your additional training in Reiki or another form of good energy transfer comes in handy. Hand holding is good if the patient seems to be comforted by it. Reading to them, humming, playing soft music for them, singing if you dare, are all sweet things to do for people with dementia or any living thing for that matter. And you can chart these activities. Invite alternative therapies if you project the patient might benefit.

Caring for patients with dementia is an art, and some people are drawn to help them. I have learned a great deal from Teepa Snow. She is a world-renowned occupational therapist who has devoted her life's work to teaching others how help those with "profound memory loss." Her entire focus is on teaching others how patients think in brain failure and how to best approach them and communicate. The enormous respect and tenderness she gives patients inspires me. I highly encourage you to read her work or at least watch her YouTube creations.

"People are precious and in the right setting can shine," Snow said. "We're not losing the person; they're still there but we need to modify our expectations and setting."[66] This is a good example of how loving and respectful Snow is. Snow says, "Instead of seeing what they lack, look at what they have. Everyone can shine in the right environment." With some of the patients with dementia I have cared for, I was able to sense their intelligence, the integrity in their life, and their kindness. I could still imagine the person despite what my eyes objectively saw or what I heard, and this helped me care for them. Seeing pictures from their past and speaking with the families is also inspiring as reminders that these were often productive and loving people.

"Your brain works better than her brain: you need to figure out how to interact—you can change the environment, the task, or your own behavior."[67] We can modify our expectations and setting.

Patients with dementia are often able to sense how we feel, so our touch and body language are cues we need to be attentive to. During a lecture,

66 "Positive Approach to Brain Change," Teepa Snow, accessed 2016, www.teepasnow.com.
67 Ibid.

Snow offered profound and important suggestions for caregivers. Smiling, walk up to the patient slowly. Try to get his or her attention with your gentle voice and hand motions before you reach the patient physically. This removes the element of surprise. Never walk up behind a patient and touch him or her. This can startle the patient. Often I have touched people before they know I am there. Snow uses an upbeat yet soft and loving tone with patients and a gentle touch. She discourages a highly stimulating atmosphere, which dementia patients struggle to interpret and may cause increased agitation. To me these patients are like newborn babies in their sensitivity and need to be treated as lovingly.

I think a PWD can smell agenda, and they will be on to you before you mention the shower you feel they must take. These cues imply "I am the boss of you," and the patient will immediately say in some form that you are not. "Quit the bossiness," Snow says. "The task is not as important as the relationship." She constantly uses praise, good humor, and respect, and the patients respond calmly to her. She is a PWD whisperer. As caregivers we tend to talk on and on about a variety of subjects, and we change subjects frequently, which makes it difficult for a PWD to follow conversations. Anxiety about silence may compel us to talk to fill in spaces. We need to keep our sentences and ideas simple and use simple visual cues.

Snow emphasizes patients are not stupid, and they pick up on subtle cues like voice tone, sounds, and the body language of frustration or anger. Snow emphasizes we must examine our anger and impatience when it arises, as it is often our own stuff being projected onto the patient.

The same principles apply to PWD: Be calm, show respect, and give up control. Look at your own issues when you feel like reacting.

CHAPTER 22

Dealing with What We Feel Is Repulsive

● ● ●

Disease and dying can be very unpretty, smelly, gooey, and noisy. Most people produce ghastly substances, especially when they are dying. I remind myself that I will too. Remembering we are all able to create the same awful smells and substances is a good equalizer.

Over time, nurses develop skills to deal with the realities of the human body and build a tolerance for it. You will come across patients with ten pounds of fourteen-hour-old urine in their Depends. Nonhealing, large, deep wounds are common in bedbound patients. Cancer, C. difficile, and infection have their own odor. Some tumors are foul smelling with weeping colorful discharge as they destroy tissue. Colostomy stomas change shape, and the appliances will not stick not matter what. Patients generally have no control over these sights and smells. There will be patients who maintain a level of hygiene we may question and judge. Some patients with poor hygiene, who we believe should be able to take better care of themselves, may no longer be aware, or are unable to smell, or they may have become desensitized to their odor. Do the task at hand efficiently with good humor. Distract the patient and yourself with pleasant conversation. Putting their feelings first will also distract you from your aversion.

Practically speaking, when I am challenged in this way, I cover body areas, body fluids, or bedpans with waterproof pads or towels. Patients are concerned and watching your reaction, so your lack of reaction is respectful.

Sometimes you will automatically and viscerally respond to certain stimulus. We all have our weak spots, so we prepare for this. You can put a dab of peppermint essential oil on your upper lip to distract your nose. It might help to be medically interested in what you are looking at. Observe tumor growth or degradation, signs of a wound healing or not, stool quality, vomit quality, for there may be important information there. Learn from each patient, so you can improve for the next. You may learn how to apply morphine bandages well on a patient with extensive tumor growth all over the side of her chest and abdomen, and you will know just what to do with the next patient who has this. You may become expert at wound packing and colostomy care, and your colleagues will be calling you to help them with their patients. Gradually, what used to repulse you will wane, or at the very least, you will learn you can get through it. If you find the task extremely distressing, you might ask to share the load with another nurse. We are guaranteed to have patients who we find physically difficult to deal with, so it benefits us to build coping skills for this.

Incontinence is inevitable, foley catheters are not. Some people are dead set against having a catheter in them, so I stick to their wishes even when they are unresponsive and it would be easier to place one. Their wishes and our respect take precedence. Of course, if their skin is deteriorating and there are wounds to consider, then I might try to discuss this with the patient and family.

CHAPTER 23

The Pillbox

● ● ●

IT REQUIRES ITS OWN CHAPTER? Yes.

Pillboxes, especially the enormous ones that hold two weeks' worth of pills with slots for four-times-a-day meds exasperate me. Those blasted pills are like Mexican jumping beans, and you will find some of Monday's tabs in Tuesday's, morning tabs in the nighttime slots. You thought you put the 2:00 p.m. seroquel in, but you did not, and metoprolol was daily, not twice daily. You realize it after you left the facility or someone calls you from the assisted-living facility and you need to return with your tail between your legs to fill it. The pillbox slots are small, and it's hard to get pills in and out, especially if your fingers are cracked and bleeding from all your documenting and handwashing, and you have several Band-Aids on. Have a good (current!) medicine list, your smallest fingers, maybe some tweezers, and try not to talk to people while you are doing the pills. People, however, really like to talk to us while we are filling the pillbox. Even without a distraction, we can make a mistake, so we must be focused. Count the meds in each slot so they all match nicely. Your eyes really can fool you, especially if you are moving quickly or the pills are the same color and shape. Take it slow filling the pillbox. Don't pull a Peggy like I did.

CHAPTER 24

Assisted-Living Facilities

● ● ●

IF YOU ARE ASSIGNED TO an ALF, find the policy for medication administration. Most likely you will need a lockbox for narcotics and sedatives and a way to document how much medicine is available daily. Some staff may be able to administer medicine only if the patient is able to take the medicine from the staff's hand without assistance. An RN must be available to administer medicines when the patient is no longer able to do this. Do not make the mistake I made one day when I had a patient in respiratory failure and could not get attention from the nursing staff or the student nurse assigned to my patient. I went to find help and found the nursing student assigned to this patient at the medicine cart. She drew up the medicine he needed, and I offered to administer it to ease her load. Which I did. Wrong. I thought I was advocating for the patient and helping the staff, but no, I was committing a near felony. It required meetings with administrators from my hospice and their facility to come to a decision on what to do with me. A real high-point in my career. I was branded and barred from the facility forever. Try to avoid this category of rejection. Hospice cannot administer medicine in a facility. Another time a facility RN was about to give a Tylenol to my patient, but then she had to run to an emergency, so she asked me to give it. I did. Woops again, but no one told the administration, so I was still able to go to that facility. The ALFs revolve around policy, procedure, and regulations. Always check in with the RN on duty that day to give and get a report on your patient.

Hospice nurses often report feeling tension between the ALF staff and their team. Understandably, ALF staff feel territorial and defensive when we come waltzing in with our ideas on how to take care of their patients. Developing as good a relationship as possible with their staff is paramount to collaborating for the patient's well-being. When we enter knowing we are their equals, they are more apt to relax with us. Communication will improve, and the job can be much more pleasant for all. Attending their staff meetings can be helpful if you can be there. Over time, once trust is established and you have proven hospice to be worthwhile and helpful, the relationships can be very good. There are times when ALFs are unyielding in their aversion for hospice staff. In these cases, you must focus on the task at hand and try not to take anything personally. Remember all Ruiz's four agreements—be impeccable with your words, do not assume anything, take nothing personally, and always do your best—work well in a setting where there are angry staff.

CHAPTER 25

Charting—Oh My

● ● ●

NURSES ARE NOW ENCOURAGED TO chart in the patients' homes. I found this a challenge because if I am charting, I am otherwise focused on the computer screen and not the patient. Personally, I am annoyed by practitioners charting during a visit. They rattle off questions and type furiously, eyes on the keyboard. One NP asked me if I ever had children, and I said no. She said, "Are you sure?" Clearly, she was not connecting to me in this moment. I prefer eye contact and to concentrate on people, not a screen. I cannot do both simultaneously. You may be more talented than I am, or your administration may command you to do it. If you must chart, do make as much eye contact as possible and focus more on the patient than the computer.

Daniel Goldman is a psychologist who speaks on compassion on NPR. He feels when we are involved face-to-face, we gain vital information that can ignite compassion, and that being engrossed in a device starves us of these clues. We lose that opportunity to act on the compassion we feel when we are charting while talking with the patient.

CHAPTER 26

Relationships with Your Own Staff

• • •

DON MIGUEL RUIZ'S FIRST AGREEMENT comes to mind when working with people, including our hospice colleagues: "Be impeccable with your word."

"Speak with integrity. Say only what you mean. Avoid using the word to speak against yourself or to gossip about others. Use the power of your in the direction of truth and love."[68] Slander will come back to the slanderer like a boomerang. Trust can be irreparably damaged. Hospice nurses need to support one another. When you hear a derogatory statement, try saying, "Wow, I find (him or her) to be observant" or whatever positive adjective fits best. People will agree with this as easily as they agreed to the damaging comments. I do wonder why it is that good comments don't usually make it around the block as fast as gossip does. Be positively creative when you want to talk behind someone's back. Make talking behind someone's back a boon to that person and to all involved.

The girl with hair on fire can be found in any workplace. She, or he, is the person who loves to inflame others with negativity and contagious gossip. She connects to others through igniting little fires. Saying something derogatory, a subtly raising an eyebrow while discussing someone, offering a little groan, or giggling condescendingly is a quick, effective strike of her match, igniting little flames that leap from one head to another. In her

---

68 Don Miguel Ruiz, *The Four Agreements.*

wake, she leaves the blazing coals of mistrust and chaos. Perhaps secretly we all love to hear others be put down because it somehow elevates us, or makes us feel safe, but I tell you, no one wins playing her game. Walk away from this sort of person, or "become like a stick of (damp) wood" as Thích Nhất Hạnh says. If you keep a cool head, her flames cannot scorch you, and if you negate her comments, you could reduce her to cool smoke.

Communicate regularly with those who share cases with you. Let them know when changes occur. Seek their counsel. I was not good at this for many years, but gradually I learned to be more inclusive. I admit to not perfecting the art of asking for assistance or working together, which was to my detriment as well as others. I think my hospice team was also having a lot more fun than I was because they had more of a sense of community. Don't do as I did. Keep the channels open.

Go to others directly when you have a concern. You might do this with a trusted supervisor or other person you respect in the office who understands this sort of nursing and the emotions involved. I was very lucky to have several wonderful, experienced nurses to whom I could take issues. Being direct builds trust.

CHAPTER 27

The Lingering Patient

● ● ●

WE LIKE TO TRY TO speculate why someone dies when he or she does, but I think that the best we can do is imagine possibilities. When a patient dies just as the prodigal son shows up, we say things like, "He waited for Johnny, that son of a gun," or "She waited until I left the room for two minutes to pee and then she died maybe because she didn't want me to see her die," or "She was able to spend Christmas with everyone and then decided to die," or "He completed his funeral arrangements and then died," Or "He waited till that grandchild was born," or a thousand other coincidences that happen close to the death. I like to guess too, and sometimes I was right on the money. I suppose I feel smart when I think I know, but I really don't know.

Sometimes people take an exceptionally long time to die, and families try to think of everything they can to nudge them along. They get the soldier home, get the funeral planned, get the estranged family member over there to visit, or get the finances finally settled. They have reassured the patient the spouse will be well cared for and the family will be OK. And the patient lives on and on and on. Everyone is exhausted. Everyone is now more than ready, and still the patient breathes in, breathes out. I speculate (see?) that those who linger stay here just long enough for loved ones to be superready for them to go, so ready that they are almost mad at them for staying. It is hard enough to say a final goodbye once. Daily goodbyes, over many weeks, exact a toll. Lingerers make for hard work

139

for the families. Don't be one when you lay dying. Support the families by giving great symptom management (of course you were already). Reiterate that people have hard work to do while they are dying, that we can't know the subconscious work they are doing, and the patient might not even be aware of this work. Elements out of our power and breadth of understanding are in control, so we must give the space and time it needs to unfold. Check exhaustion levels daily. Offer increased team support.

CHAPTER 28

Postmortem Care

● ● ●

AFTER A PATIENT DIES, I have learned to offer certain things that families have told me were very helpful. After I listen with my stethescope and make the official pronouncement that the heart has stopped, I call the team. I may clean up the patient or room just a bit. I position myself in the background or the perimeter of the room so that the family can gather together. Encourage people to come and go to the bedside if they desire. I ask if, and when, they would like me to wash to body. Occasionally caregivers ask that the patient remain as he or she is. Often more family will be arriving, so I try to have the patient and the room ready for visitors. I play a low-key, task-oriented role while keeping an eye on who needs more personal support.

I tell people that there is no rush to accomplish anything. I call the funeral home to give basic information. I ask the funeral home staff to wait for the family to be ready for them to pick up their loved one. Sometimes families want the funeral home to come quickly, other times they may want to wait many hours for other family members to come. Then again, the funeral home may not be able to be there for hours. If there will be more than a few hours of waiting, I am careful to describe to the family what they can expect to see from the body, such as color changes and possible expelling of air, urine, and feces.

While giving the bath, I invite others to be there or even assist. Some start and cannot finish and some enter later. Family members have told me that assisting with the bath was a peaceful, lovely way to spend a bit more time with their loved one. Another spouse deeply regretted not being there and even mentioned it to me many months later as her one regret. This last bath is important for most people, even to you, the nurse. It confers dignity and respect to the patient and family for all they have gone through. It may be the last time families will touch this person or see him or her, and this last hour or two with the person will be firmly implanted in their memories. Then again, it is OK if they have no contact with the body because they may be too overwhelmed.

If there is a friend or family member that wishes to assist with the final bath, explain what it may feel like in terms of weight and temperature. Encourage the family to pick out the clothes for the funeral home, for transport, and then for the funeral. It is quite difficult to dress a woman in nylons/bras/underwear/skirt and tight sweater and men in jeans and button-down shirts, but if this is what the family requests, it must be attempted. Wash the body with warm water and use soap. Keep the body covered in blankets or a towel as many times family have mentioned that their loved one might be cold. You could ask for their favorite perfume or cologne and use lightly. I once put Old Spice on a deceased female patient because it was her deceased husband's favorite and she loved it and often wore it herself. The family loved this. Put Depends on if you can because of the sphincter relaxation that can occur. Most families like clean socks to be put on their loved ones. Shave the patient as needed. Families love this too. Place their rosaries in their hands if this feels right to the family. I have put other sentimental items in patients' hands, such as another religious item, a small picture, a flower, and for one patient with dementia, I put about ten of his favorite small stuffed animals on the bed with him. I have put Red Sox or Patriot hats and other paraphernalia on many. Make it personal.

Be very gentle with the body. Hum something sweet. Your careful and slow manner shows respect. Consider how you would like others to treat your body, or that of your loved one, at death. Working alone with a large dead body is strenuous, and you might not appear gentle as you use your brute strength to move a body side to side to clean and dress them, so try to have privacy. Just do your best. Sometimes it is just too difficult to get tight jeans on a large body, and you may have to be honest with the family about this. Sweats and shirts cut up the back are much easier, and you can ask for this if you feel the timing is right.

When possible, stay with the family until the funeral home staff arrive. The family finds this helpful. You have time to tidy the room, discard medicine, attend to those who need attending, and call others to alert of death. Discard medical tubing. Make sure the patient and bedding looks organized and clean. You can gently guide the conversation if need be and cajole folks into reminiscing, but more often they are able to do this without your input. Should the family wish to have the body picked up later, it may be fine to leave, but do check in with them later to make sure everything went according to plan and that they are OK. These last few hours you spend with the patient and family are meaningful, and it is good closure for all. Take your time and try to keep your schedule off your mind. Call the office and let them know you are tied up. Rarely did I absolutely need to leave a pronouncement, but the few times it happened I felt badly, like I was shortchanging the family.

Don't forget to leave the perfectly complete pronouncement form for the funeral home. Bring a few along. It only takes one miniscule mistake for the funeral home to reject it.

Once the body has been removed, further tidy the room and clean up the linen. Often, I start the laundry to spare the family the task of seeing soiled sheets. Ask what articles they would like to keep. Get rid of all the mouth swabs, cloudy water, syringes. Ask what they would like to do with extra Depends, cloth pads, and so forth. You could casually mention that your hospice's patients could really use those cloth pads and extra Depends.

Leave the family with telephone numbers for follow up. Remind them that the hospice bereavement service will be calling soon.

Leaving is very hard, and there is no easy way to do it. It's just awkward, especially if you know them, but also if you don't know them! If you've had a wonderful experience with the family and feel the love, you might say, "See you at the service." If I don't know them, I ask if there is anything else I can do for them or anyone I can call. I encourage them to call us with concerns. After a few days or weeks questions develop, especially concerning the actual death. The family may worry and say things like "Do you think he died peacefully," or "I don't think he died well." Families can torture themselves with these questions. and their grief will be more difficult if these concerns are not addressed.

It's just plain hard to break ties with people without offering ungenuine comments, such as "We will be in touch." You probably will not be, so do not offer anything that cannot be followed through on.

I have found for the most part that once the experience with a family is complete, I quietly close the door and walk away. I am surprised how easily I can do this, especially if I have enjoyed and connected well with the patient and family and loved being with them. Although it is hard to initially break the tie, to close the door the last time, over the long haul, I find it drifts naturally away, and it becomes harder for me to reopen the door. Invariably, I will be admitting a new family very soon, maybe even that day, so being busy can soften the loss.

Our hospice invites families who have lost someone to a memorial service annually. I go, but I squirm through this ceremony no matter how much

I loved my patients and families. Embarrassingly and surprisingly, I may not even recognize the family out of context. Memories will return with prompting, but I find I let go of most of these experiences. The tide comes in and gently washes away our footprints. I do not see this as bad or sad but as a natural and necessary letting go. I believe our task in life is to learn to let go. Hospice nursing certainly will offer this opportunity.

CHAPTER 29

Burnout—Me?

● ● ●

YOU MAY HAVE TIMES WHEN your hospice work feels overwhelming and you feel exhausted, depleted, and frustrated. You may feel like you can't do it any longer, or you are not cut out for hospice nursing. I cannot say whether this is true for you or not, but some people realize they cannot do this work. Before you make any change, it is important to investigate your feelings. A wonderful therapist friend of mine encourages us to look for the leaks in our boats. We may appear to be floating, in control, and high-functioning, yet when we peer beneath the vessel, we find small, or not so small, leaks in our structures, in our awareness. Our energy sneaks out, and little by little we start to sink. The leaks may be due to poor self-care, self-doubts, anger, or jealousy. These emotions and reactions need attending to for our survival.

Jean Watson said burnout occurs "not because we care too much, but because we wall ourselves off, close off our heart, close off our source of love and the human connectedness that gives us life generating force for this work."[69] It is important to examine your pain and perhaps your anger. Have you disconnected from your patients and colleagues? Communicating with a trusted supervisor or friend may be very helpful. I was always very fortunate to have fantastic administration who listened to my doubts and questions.

---

69 Watson, *Care for the Journey.*

Ask what sustains you, regenerates you, and heals you aside from work. It will be critical for you to find replenishment. For each of us it is different, but find something that feeds your soul. That could be simply sitting on the couch petting your peaceful cat. There are as many ways to find rejuvenation as there are people in the world.

Cate Stillman writes, "Right behind the facade of stress is the subtle backdrop of expanded awareness. Under your insecurities is your competency. The stress mindset causes you to forget you are whole, that you are A-OK in this moment. You compete, not collaborate. You construct obstacles instead of creating solutions. Yet, our expanded awareness is always right here, not even a breath away."[70] If we remember this higher thinking when we are in the throes of frustration, disillusionment, or disconnection, perhaps fewer nurses would experience burnout.

---

70 Stillman, *Body Thrive*, 242.

EPILOGUE

● ● ●

SINCE COMPLETING THIS BOOK, I have retired from hospice nursing. It was not a case of burnout, but rather a desire to go into a new field of caring for others. I heard the call to leave for a while before I gave notice. It was not sudden or out of anger or anything negative. It was just my time to go. My years in hospice were rewarding and a highlight in my nursing career. I believe strongly in the worth of hospice, the beauty of being with people, of standing quietly with them under the waterfall, sometimes next to them, sometimes a bit to the side, but firmly with them as they navigate this natural flow of life and death.

If I am fortunate enough to have time for hospice at the end of my life, I want hospice nurses strong enough to let me run the show if I want to. I hope they can make me laugh, open my heart to insights, take a read on my family so they know how best to support them, and remind me of God. I hope this nurse can walk away from my home on that my last day and be grateful for the experience of my family, as I so often felt.

It was a daily reminder goodness abounds.

The patients and families I was lucky enough to be with enriched my life immeasurably. I thank each of them. I will miss the depth of these relationships, the banter, the laughing and crying, and the learning. I loved the intensity of working with people who know they are dying. They never failed to remind me that goodness abounds.

I feel very honored to have been called to hospice nursing.

Here is a little reminder from Desmond Tutu about how important your work is and how valuable you are even without your work:

> Your preciousness cannot be computed. Nothing can separate you from the source of all life. Nothing, not disease, suffering, not even death. Remember what brought you here in the first place. You were born to uplift and help others. Have mercy! Please be kind to yourself. We are, after, all just human, which is good enough. Go forth sustained by the knowledge you are precious, embraced, able to go forth with a courage that is not your own because its source is the source of all that is beautiful, that is good, that is true![71]

Always remember that you are connected to a great source that will show you how to love in your unique way and will bless you into usefulness.

---

71 M. Stillwater and Gary Malkin, Desmond Tutu in *Care for the Journey*, Companion Arts, 2005, CD-ROM #TK.

REFERENCES

Bronwen and Frans Stiene. *The Reiki Sourcebook*. UK: O Books, 2008.

Byock, Ira, MD. *Dying Well*. New York: Riverhead Books, 1997.

Care for the Journey: Messages and Music for Sustaining the Heart of Healing. Companion Arts in association with Wisdom of the World. Boulder, CO: Companion Arts, 2015. CD-ROM. www.companionarts.org

Douglass, Frederick. *Daily Calm 365 Days of Serenity*. Washington, DC: National Geographic, 2013.

Earl, Ester. *This Star Won't Go Out*. New York: Dutton, 2014.

Gawande, Atul, MD. *Being Mortal: Medicine and What Matters in the End*. New York: Henry Holt and Company, 2014.

Gawande, Atul, MD. "Letting Go. What Should Medicine Do When It Can't Save Your Life?" *The New Yorker*, August 2, 2010.

Goldberg, Natalie. *Long Quiet Highway: Waking Up in America*. New York and London: Bantam, 1993

Hanh, Thich Nhat. "Mindfulness of Breathing." Dharma Talk. July 24, 1998.

Hanh, Thich Nhat. *Peace Is Every Step: The Path of Mindfulness in Everyday Life*. New York: Bantam, 1992. Hanh, Thich Nhat. *Your True Home: The Everyday Wisdom of Thich Nhat Hanh: 365 Days of Practical, Powerful Teachings from the Beloved Zen Teacher*. Boulder, CO: Shambhala Publications, 2011.

Kabat-Zinn, J. and M. Kabat-Zinn. *Everyday Blessings*. New York: Hyperion, 1998.

Paramananda, Swami. *Book of Daily Thoughts and Prayers.* Cohasset, MA: Vedanta Center Publishers, 1977.

Rinpoche, Sogyal. *The Tibetan Book of Living and Dying.* San Francisco: Harper, 1993.

Ruiz, Don Miguel. *The Four Agreements: A Practical Guide to Personal Freedom.* San Rafael, CA: Amber Allen Publishing

Rinpoche, Sogyal. *The Tibetan Book of Living and Dying.* San Francisco: Harper, 1993.

Ruiz, Don Miguel. *The Four Agreements: A Practical Guide to Personal Freedom.* San Rafael, CA: Amber Allen Publishing, 1997.

Singh, S. *Spiritual Gems.* Punjab, India: Radha Soami Satsang Beas, 2007.

Stillman, Cate. *Body Thrive.* Tetonia, ID: Yoga Healer Press, 2015.

Ueshiba, Morihei. *The Art of Peace*, translated and edited by John Stevens. Boulder, CO: Shambhala Publications, Inc., 2002.

Watson, Jean. "Intentionality and Caring-Healing Consciousness: A Practice of Transpersonal Nursing." *Holistic Nursing Practice* 16, no. 4 (2002): 12–19.

Welch, Claudia, DOM. *How the Art of Medicine Makes the Science More Effective Becoming the Medicine We Practice.* London and Philadelphia: Singing Dragon, 2015.

Zucker, Deborah, ND. *The Vitality Map: A Guide to Deep Health, Joyful Self-Care, and Resilient Well-Being. LomaSerena Press,* 2016.

APPENDIX A: MINDFULNESS
OF BREATHING

● ● ●

"WE HAVE TO LEARN HOW to rest. Deep relaxation here is one of the methods of resting. Sitting meditation is another means to rest. In order to rest, we have to know how to use our breathing.

The first exercise that the Buddha proposed is "While I am breathing in, I am aware that this is breathing in; and I breathe out, and I am aware that I am breathing out. Recognizing breathing in as breathing in, and breathing out as breathing out.

Second exercise: I breathe in and I am aware of the length of my in-breath; breathing out, I am aware of the length of my out-breath. We become aware of the length of the in-breath and the out-breath.

Third exercise: I breathe in, and I am aware of my whole body. We recognize our whole body being present here, either sitting, lying down, standing or walking. Breathing is to generate the object of mindfulness.

Fourth exercise: Breathing in, I calm the activities of my physical body. My physical body, I am here for you. Take care, be interested in your physical body, and start to take care of your physical body. Become aware of different parts of your body. "I breathe in, I am aware of my eyes, I breathe out, and I smile to my eyes."[72]

---

72 "Mindfulness of Breathing" from Dharma Talk given by Thích Nhất Hạnh on July 24th, 1998, in Plum Village, France.

APPENDIX B: BREATH WORK

● ● ●

ALTERNATE NOSTRIL BREATHING:

Sit comfortably with your back straight and eyes closed. Fold the first and second fingers of your right hand into your palm.

Close off your right nostril with your right thumb. Inhale through the left nostril. Close your left nostril with the ring finger of your right hand and retain the breath briefly and gently. Open your right nostril by removing your right thumb and exhale.

With left hand still closed, inhale through the right nostril. Close off the right nostril with your thumb. Retain the breath briefly. Then open your left nostril by removing your ring finger and exhale.

Repeat this process for up to fifteen minutes, but even doing it five times is a benefit.

Three-Part Breath:

This can be done either lying down or sitting up. As you slowly inhale through your nose, inflate first the abdomen, then feel the rib cage expand outward, then feel the clavicles rise as you fully inflate your lungs. On the exhale deflate the lungs slowly, being aware of the clavicles moving down, the rib cage softly moving in, and the abdomen moving back toward the spine. Repeat at least five times. This is a deeply restful breath.

APPENDIX C: TIPS FOR SITTING IN SILENCE

● ● ●

START WITH ONE MINUTE DEEP breathing practice.

Bring 100 percent awareness to this one-minute practice. Try it before sleep or in the early morning.

Sit in the same place every time you practice.

Use an audio recording if needed.

Set the timer on your phone and stick with the one minute. Gradually increase. Work your way up. Consistency is more important than duration.

Commit to daily practice.

Bring your focus back to simply paying attention when it drifts. And it will—constantly, at first.

Use a meditation app if desired.

Find other meditators.[73]

---

73 Stillman, Body Thrive. 196.

APPENDIX D
FAQ'S ABOUT HOSPICE

● ● ●

Is it true when people come on hospice they die right away?

Some people die within days of being on hospice, but the average stay on hospice is about two months. Each persons' disease process is different so there is no standard. Your doctor needs to be able to document for insurance purposes, that he would not be surprised if you died within six months. People can remain on hospice for as long as they meet certain criteria. There must be measurable signs of decline, such as significant weight loss, need for symptom management, severe weakness, and confusion or agitation. It is helpful to come on hospice as soon as one meets criteria to benefit from the holistic services. Unfortunately, some patients come to hospice late, needlessly suffering from less than optimal symptom management and inadequate physical and emotional support for the family.

Do I have to take morphine?

Hospice nurses do not force you to do anything against your will. An in-depth discussion of your feelings about morphine will help clarify its uses and benefits. Morphine is an effective pain medicine for many types of pain. Certain diseases cause pain that requires a stronger medicine than Tylenol or Motrin. Most patients experience great relief from morphine and only a few do not tolerate it. In hospice meds are given slowly and at a low dose to begin, and then are increased as the patient tolerates or needs more. If morphine does not make a patient feel better, other medicine will be offered by the doctor.

If you are comfortable, you can enjoy your family and friends during this important time. Taking even small doses of medicine benefits you and others.

Will I be over-dosed on medicine while on hospice care?

Hospice nurses do not over-dose patients. The patient can choose how they wish to feel. One patient may wish to have less medicine, be more alert, and accept some level of pain, while another may wish to be a bit sleepy, but experience less pain. Sometimes, patients need a great deal of medicine to be comfortable, which can cause them to feel drowsy. Medicine is for comfort. The goal of hospice care is physical and emotional comfort. When a patient reaches their goal for comfort the medicine can be kept at the dose that achieves that level. Nurses will discuss this on admission and evaluate pain levels during each visit. Palliative sedation, is a deeper form of sedation a patient or family chooses when symptoms have become unbearable. This is discussed at length between the patient, family, and doctor prior to giving the medicine. The *intention* in palliative sedation is to provide comfort, even if the dose eventually could be cause death.

What happens if I do not meet criteria while on hospice?

There are certification periods in hospice care. Medicare has two ninety day periods and sixty day periods after that. Toward the end of the benefit period the nurse and possibly the doctor will evaluate a patient's condition and discuss why the patient qualifies or not. A discharge should not come as a surprise to the patient or family. If discharge seems likely, patients and families are prepared in advance and options for services outside of hospice are offered. Some patients and families will not feel happy about being discharged and losing hospice services. They have the option to appeal the decision. The good news is that the patient can come back on hospice as soon as criteria can be met. This could even be the next day if their status changes.

A patient can revoke hospice services as well if they decide they would like to seek rehabilitation or curative procedures. I have heard people say, after being on hospice, they dislike the implications of being on hospice and will then opt out of care. There is no right or wrong way to do this. People come to hospice when they are ready and leave if they wish.

Can I have the same nurse all the time?

Hospice staff hopes for continuity, but it is hard to work every day. The hospice agency will try their hardest to have a consistent team of nurses, home health aides, social workers, chaplain and volunteers. Even with best efforts this is difficult because of the ever-changing nature of patients and staffs' status. Luckily, the team documents on computers shared by team members so information is (usually) current.

What does hospice cost?

Hospice services include nursing, home health aides, social workers, chaplain, and volunteers. These are covered under the hospice benefit on your insurance or Medicare.

Your insurance plan must be approved by the hospice agency.

Medicine related to your diagnosis will be covered. The doctor decides this immediately following the admission.

Equipment related to your disease is also covered, such as, wheelchairs, commodes, walkers, nebulizers, hospital beds, special mattresses (if the patient meets criteria for this).

How will I be treated after I die?

Gently and with utmost care and respect. Families are present and often wish to help with bathing and dressing a body. These final moments are considered sacred by many hospice nurses.

Can hospice go in nursing homes, assisted living facilities and hospitals?

Yes. Hospice staff becomes adjunct staff to these facilities. We assist with symptom management and offer support to staff through the team.

What if I don't want all those people from hospice in my home?

It is not mandatory for a patient to receive all the services other than nursing and one social worker visit. The insurance companies must have a nurses' documentation of the patients' condition every two weeks, minimum. The staff spaces visits so the family and patient do not feel overwhelmed by frequent visits. They also try to accommodate the families' schedule.

Can I keep my doctor?

Yes. Generally, your primary care doctor, or the referring doctor, stays involved. They write your orders while you are on hospice. Hospices have a medical director who can write your orders if your doctor is unavailable or that doctor requests the medical director to help with your symptom management.

Will you remember me after I am gone?

Yes. You can rest assured you made an indelible imprint on those who cared for you. I am sure I speak for many saying, we are grateful.

I love this quote of Natalie Goldberg's.

> Whether we know it or not, we transmit the presence of everyone
> we have ever known, as though by being in each other's presence
> we exchange our cells, pass on some of our life force, and then we
> go on carrying that other person in our body, not unlike spring-
> time when certain plants in fields we walk through attach their
> seeds tin the form of small burrs to our socks, our pants, our caps,
> as if to say, "Go on, take us with you, carry us to root in another
> place."

Natalie Goldberg. *Long Quiet Highway: Waking Up in America*, (New York
and London: Bantam, 1993), 74.